RESEARCH AND PERSPECTIVES IN LONGEVITY

J.R. Carey J.-M. Robine
J.-P. Michel Y. Christen (Eds.)

# Longevity and Frailty

With 36 Figures and 12 Tables

Springer

*James R. Carey*, Ph.D.
Department of Entomology
University of California
One Shields Ave.
Davis, CA 95616
USA
e-mail: Jrcarey@ucdavis.edu

*Jean Pierre Michel*, MD
Département de Gériatrie
HUG
Route de Mon Idée
1226 Thonex
Switzerland
E-mail: Jean-pierre.michel@hcuge.ch

*Jean-Marie Robine*, Ph.D.
CRLC, Val d'Aurelle
INSERM Equipe Démographie et Santé
Parc Euromédecine
34298 Montpellier Cedex 05
France
E-mail: robine@valdorel.fnclcc.fr

*Yves Christen*, Ph.D.
Fondation IPSEN
Pour la Recherche Thérapeutique
24, rue Erlanger
75781 Paris Cedex 16
France
e-mail: yves.christen@beaufour-ipsen.com

ISBN 3-540-25153-7 Springer-Verlag Berlin Heidelberg New York

Library of Congress Control Number: 2005921468



Springer-Verlag is a part of Springer Science+Business Media

springeronline.com


Printed in Germany



Editor: Dr. Rolf Lange, Heidelberg
Desk Editor: Anne Clauss, Heidelberg
Production: PRO EDIT GmbH, 69126 Heidelberg, Germany
Cover design: design & production, 69121 Heidelberg, Germany
Typesetting: SDS, Leimen, Germany
Printed on acid-free paper 27/3150Re – 5 4 3 2 1 0

# Preface

Frailty is a transitional state between robustness and physical dependency and indeed lead to increase mortality. This concept is central to the study of longevity because the frailty status of individuals is used as a proxy for both their aging rate and mortality risk, models of frailty provide important insights into mortality change, frailty indices are used for investigations of active life span and successful aging, clinical studies on frailty shed light on the etiology of impairment and the physiology of aging, and experimental research on frailty in model organisms provides important insights into the molecular and genetic bases of disablement. The 13 papers that follow draw on many of these concepts and are the outcome of the interdisciplinary colloquium "Longevity and Frailty" held in Paris in October of 2004 and sponsored by Fondation IPSEN. One of the animating concepts for the meeting was to bring together a mixture of researchers with diverse backgrounds and perspectives on aging, frailty and longevity including experimental biologists, geriatricians, human biologists/anthropologists and demographers.

The first four papers are concerned with research on each of four different animal models including the medfly used for studying frailty and active life expectancy (Carey and Papadopoulos), the honey bee used to demonstrate that the plasticity of aging emerges through an interplay between a systemic hormone and a gene normally expressed by reproductive females (Amdam), the nematode used to reveal that the insulin/IGF-1 pathway ultimately exerts its effect on life span by up-regulating a wide variety of genes (Murphy), and the rhesus monkey used in long-term studies to show that the effects of calorie restriction (CR) have a positive influence on frailty and longevity (Ingram and colleagues).

The next series of four papers involve evolutionary, conceptual, physiological, and molecular sub-themes including an overview of frailty in hominids and a reiteration of the importance of perspectives on frailty derived from evolutionary medicine (Crews). For example, inflammation plays an important role in the genesis of the frailty syndrome but inflammation itself is an evolutionary defense against infection (Ferrucci and colleagues), disability processes in long-lived animals may be similar to those in humans and thus serve as models for studying processes disablement (Verbrugge), biological markers such as muscle weakness may be used in conjunction with molecular triggering mechanisms for inflammation to understand the etiology of frailty (Waltson), and frailty and cognition appear to be inextricably intertwined (Michel and colleagues). A reduction in the extent and time spent with high levels of inflammatory markers may have been part of a physiological revolution that accounted for the decrease in mortality at young ages which occurred when infectious diseases were reduced last century in developed countries (Crimmins and Finch).

Evidence of morbidity compression – a manifestation of reductions in the incidence of frailty relative to the incidence of mortality – is reflected in the recent finding that U.S. population is experiencing a 2% annual reduction in disability rates but a 1% decline in mortality rates (Fries). However, the consequences of the ever-increasing prevalence of frailty due to aging populations are reflected in the large increase in heat-related deaths in France during an exceptional heatwave in August 2003 (Jougla and Hémon) and projections of the prevalence of long term care needs for the oldest old in developed countries based on time series projections (Robine). It is not clear yet whether the world is accumulating healthy elderly or frail oldest-old.

## Acknowledgement

The editors want to thank Jacqueline Mervaillie for the organization of the meeting and Mary Lynn Gage and Astrid de Gérard for the editing of the book.

February 2005

*James R. Carey*
*Jean-Marie Robine*
*Jean-Pierre Michel*
*Yves Christen*

# Contents

# Contributors

*Amdam, Gro V.*
Department of Entomology, University of California, Davis, 95616 CA, USA
and
Department of Animal Science, Agricultural University of Norway, 1432 Aas, Norway

*Anson, Michael R.*
Laboratory of Experimental Gerontology, Gerontology Research Center, National Institute on Aging, National Institute of Health, 5600 Nathan Shock Drive, Baltimore, MD 21224
USA

*Bandinelli Stefania, MD*
INRCA, Florence, Italy

*Ble, Alessandro, MD*
National Institute on Aging, Clinical Research Branch, Harbor Hospital Center, Room NM-534, 5th Floor, 3001 S.Hanover St., Baltimore MD 21225
USA

*Bonin-Guillaume, S.*
Département de Réhabilitation et Gériatrie, Hôpitaux Universitaires de Genève, Université de Genève, 3, chemin du Pont-Bochet, 1226 Thônex-Genève, Switzerland

*Carey, James R.*
Department of Entomology, University of California, One Shields Ave., Davis, CA 95616,
USA

*Crews, Douglas E.*
Department of Anthropology and School of Public Health, The Ohio State University, 244 Lord Hall, 124 W. 17th Ave., Colombus, OH 43210-1364
USA

*Crimmins, Eileen M.*
Andrus Gerontology Center, University of Southern California,
Suite 218D, 3715 McClintock Avenue, Los Angeles, CA 90089-0191,
USA

*de Cabo, Rafael*
Laboratory of Experimental Gerontology, Gerontology Research Center,
National Institute on Aging, National Institute of Health,
5600 Nathan Shock Drive, Baltimore, MD 21224
USA

*Finch, Caleb E.*
Andrus Gerontology Center, University of Southern California,
Suite 218D, 3715 McClintock Avenue, Los Angeles, CA 90089-0191,
USA

*Ferrucci, Luigi*
National Institute on Aging, Clinical Research Branch, Harbor Hospital Center,
Room NM-534, 5th Floor, 3001 S.Hanover St., Baltimore MD 21225,
USA

*Fries, James F.*
Department of Medicine, Stanford University School of Medicine, Stanford,
CA 94304, Palo Alto California,
USA

*Gold, Gabriel*
Département de Réhabilitation et Gériatrie, Hôpitaux Universitaires de Genève,
Université de Genève, Genève,
Switzerland

*Hémon, Denis*
INSERM-U170 -IFR 69,
Recherches épidémiologiques et statistiques sur l'environnement et la santé,
Villejuif,
France

*Herrmann, François*
Département de Réhabilitation et Gériatrie, Hôpitaux Universitaires de Genève,
Université de Genève, 3, chemin du Pont-Bochet, 1226 Thônex-Genève,
Switzerland

*Ingram, Donald K.*
Laboratory of Experimental Gerontology, Gerontology Research Center,
National Institute on Aging, NIH, 5600 Nathan Shock Drive, Baltimore,
MD 21224,
USA

*Jougla, Eric*
INSERM-CépiDc -IFR 69,
Centre d'Epidémiologie sur les causes médicales de décès,
44, Chemin de Ronde, Bât D, 78116 Le Vésinet Cedex,
France

*Lane, Mark A.*
Merck and Company, 126 E Lincoln Ave., Rahway, NJ 07065,
USA

*Mattison, Julie A.*
Laboratory of Experimental Gerontology, Gerontology Research Center,
National Institute on Aging, National Institute of Health,
5600 Nathan Shock Drive, Baltimore, MD 21224,
USA

*Michel, Jean-Pierre*
Département de Réhabilitation et Gériatrie,
Hôpitaux Universitaires de Genève - Université de Genève,
Centre Interfacultaire de Gérontologie - Université de Genève,
3, chemin du Pont-Bochet - 1226 Thônex-Genève,
Switzerland

*Murphy, Coleen T.*
University of California, Mission Bay, 600 16th St. GH-S314, San Francisco,
CA 94158
USA

*Ottinger, Mary Ann*
Department of Avian and Animal Science, University of Maryland,
College Park, MD 20742,
USA

*Papadopoulos, Nikos*
University Thessaly, Department of Agriculture Crop Production and
Rural Environment, Laboratory of Entomology and Applied Zoology,
Phytokou St. N. 384 46 N. Ionia Magnisias, Volos,
Greece

*Robine, Jean-Marie*
Inserm, Démographie et Santé, CRLC & Université de Montpellier 1,
Val d´Aurelle, Parc Euromédecine, 34298 Montpellier Cedex 05,
France

*Roth, George S.*
Laboratory of Experimental Gerontology, Gerontology Research Center,
National Institute on Aging, National Institute of Health,
5600 Nathan Shock Drive, Baltimore, MD 21224,
USA

*Simonsick, Eleanor M., PhD*
National Institute on Aging, Clinical Research Branch,
Harbor Hospital Center, Room NM-534, 5th Floor,
3001 S.Hanover St., Baltimore MD 21225,
USA

*Verbrugge, Lois M.*
Asia Research Institute, Shaw foundation Bldg., Block AS7, Level 4,
5 Arts Link, National University of Singapore, Singapore 117570,
and
University of Michigan, Institute of Gerontology, 300 N. Ingalls,
Ann Arbor MI 48109-2007,
USA

*Walston, Jeremy D., MD*
Division of Geriatric Medicine and Gerontology,
Johns Hopkins University School of Medicine, JHAAC Rm. 5A.24,
5505 Bayview Circle, Baltimore, MD 21224,
USA

*Windham, B. Gwen, MD, M.H.S*
National Institute on Aging, Clinical Research Branch, Harbor Hospital Center,
Room NM-534, 5th Floor, 3001 S.Hanover St., Baltimore MD 21225,
USA

# The Medfly as a Frailty Model: Implications for Biodemographic Research

*James R. Carey*[1] *and Nikos Papadopoulos*[2]

## Summary

Despite the economic, medical and demographic importance of understanding the determinants of chronic disability and frailty in particular and morbidity compression in general, the experimental method and model (animal) systems have not been brought to bear on questions related to these areas. Thus the purpose of this paper is to 1) briefly review the basic concepts of disability and impairment as they relate to both humans and non-human animals. 2) present the results of a study of medflies in which individuals can be classified as healthy or unhealthy based on whether they exhibit "supine behavior," and 3) introduce a general framework for research on morbidity that integrates experimental biology (manipulative experiments, model animals, hypothesis testing) into the current clinically based morbidity research paradigm on humans.

## Introduction

Chronic disability in general and degenerative diseases in particular are considered by the biomedical and public health establishments to be the most important (and costly) issues in health care confronting developed countries such as the US and France in the 21$^{st}$ century. For example, chronic diseases with limitations on activity affect as much as 10% of the US population, primarily among the elderly (Lollar and Crews 2003). This percentage will continue to increase because the number of individuals in the US over age 65 is predicted to double from 35 million in 2000 to an estimated 70 million in 2030 (Mehrotra et al. 2002). With health care costs already accounting for 15% ($1.5 trillion) of the US economy (Mehrotra et al. 2002), this surge in the elderly population will increase this percentage even further, because health care costs for those over 65 average three times the costs for those aged 19 to 65.

[1] Department of Entomology, University of California, Davis, CA 95616; and Center for the Economics and Demography of Aging, University of California, Berkeley 94720 USA

[2] University Thessaly, Department of Agriculture Crop Production and Rural Environment, Laboratory of Entomology and Applied Zoology Phytokou St. N. 384 46 N. Ionia Magnisias, Volos, Greece

Carey et al.
Longevity and Frailty

Understanding chronic disability is important for several reasons (Manton et al. 1997). First, as life expectancy continues to increase, it is important to understand if and to what extent disabilities will increase. This information will shed important light on the period of life spent disabled, which, in turn, has profound implications regarding the cost of Social Security and the debate over retirement age. For example, a relative rate of improvement of 1.5% per annum in chronic disability could ensure the long-term fiscal solvency of the Medicare and Social Security programs (Singer and Manton 1998). Second, because chronic disability is a sensitive measure of age-related changes in the health and biological fitness of individuals, disability is a marker of whether life expectancy increases are associated with changes in the age rate of the loss of the average biological fitness of a population (i.e., marker of biological rate of aging). Third, increases in birth rates and in-migration cannot be counted upon to replace losses to the stock of human capital available in the U S economy. Thus the only viable strategy is to adopt programs that will preserve human capital and keep it in the labor force for longer periods of time (Manton and Gu 2001).

Clearly, health and health care expenditures in developed countries for the 21st century must be based on a strategy designed to develop new conceptual and practical approaches for health and solid theoretical and empirical foundations for considering research policy on disablement. Despite the statement a decade ago by Verbrugge and Jette ( 1994) that "...there is great need for more theoretical work about how onset and duration affect the disablement experience," there has been little progress on either theory or empirical data. We believe a large reason for this lack of progress is the absence of an experimental research paradigm. For example, neither of the "bibles" on disability - the 850-page *Handbook of Disability Studies* (Albrecht et al. 2001) and the 300-page WHO-publication *International Classification of Functioning, Disability and Health* (WHO 2001) - contains any reference to the experimental biology literature.

There are several reasons why the experimental method has not been brought to bear on questions concerning frailty and disablement processes. First, no model system has been developed for studying the dynamics of impairment and disability. Aging research focuses on death as the endpoint rather than on the onset of impairment or chronic disease. Second, the same types of problems of ambiguity arise in characterizing disablement and morbidity in model systems as with humans. That is, unlike the (usually) unambiguous endpoint of death, in the vast majority of cases the endpoint of active life span (i.e., onset of chronic disease and/or impairment) is subjective and arbitrary, involving composite scores on a battery of Activities of Daily Living indices (ADLs). Third, just as actuarial studies of mortality require the use of large initial numbers to measure patterns at older ages, investigations on morbidity also require large numbers, particularly for studies concerned with the interrelationship of morbidity and mortality.

We have two main goals in this paper ; first, to describe the results of a study by Papadopoulos and co-workers (Papadopoulos et al. 2002, 2004) in which a new and unique behavior, referred to as "supine behavior" was discovered in older medfly males that serves as a biomarker for deteriorating health and impending death. We use this study as a foundation upon which more general concepts are built, including the development of a simple model to explore the effects of changes in hazard rates on life expectancy and morbidity compression; and second, to discuss the general implications for the use of insect models in particular and animal models more generally to research the dynamics of morbidity and mortality. We argue that the development of a broader and more basic paradigm that includes experimental methods and the use of a model is critical for advancing an understanding of the biology and demography of morbidity.

## Biodemography of frailty in medflies

### Background

A biomarker of aging is a behavioral or biological parameter of an organism that either alone or in some multivariate composite will better predict functional capacity and/or mortality risk at some late age than chronological age will (Markowska and Breckler 1999; Papadopoulos et al. 2002). Behavior biomarkers of aging are important because 1) behavior changes with aging and thus behavior itself can be used as an index of aging, and 2) any intervention to alter the chronological course of aging must be assessed behaviorally since quality of life as well as longevity must be considered in the evaluation of any intervention (Baker and Sprott 1988). Because of their rapid generation time and low cost relative to mammalian models such as rodents or primates, understanding behavioral biomarkers in fruit flies has important implications for research designed to understand morbidity dynamics, behavioral neuroethology and gerontology, and the interpretation of longevity extension in model organisms.

While monitoring the behavior of male Mediterranean fruit flies (*Ceratitis capitata*) throughout their lives, Papadopoulos and co-workers (2002) discovered a behavioral trait that is unique to older, geriatric flies in general but especially to individuals that are gradually approaching death. They used the term supine behavior to describe this behavior trait in accordance with the upside-down position of the temporarily immobile flies (Fig. 1). Supine males lie on their backs at the bottom of the cage, appearing dead or moribund. But these flies are very much alive and moderately robust, as becomes evident when they right themselves either spontaneously or after gentle prodding and initiate walking, eating, and wing-fanning behaviors, some of which are indistinguishable from those of normal flies.

Inasmuch as any upside-down adult insect is dysfunctional, it follows that the health of medfly males that we observed spending progressively greater amounts of time in the supine position was both poor and declining relative to the health of flies capable of remaining upright. Because virtually nothing is known about the nature of chronic conditions (illnesses, infirmity, dementia) in insects, as no viable animal model systems exist for studying morbidity dynamics (e.g., determinants, age of onset, persistence, association with mortality), and because of the importance of understanding morbidity incidence and prevalence in human populations, we initiated studies designed to address and test a number of questions regarding supine behavior in medfly males: When do flies first begin to exhibit supine behavior? Is it sporadic or progressive? What is the age and frequency

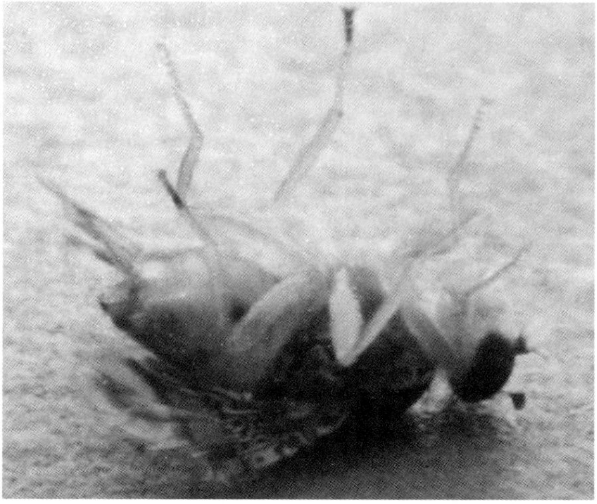

**Fig. 1.** Male Mediterranean fruit fly male in supine position. When supine flies are disturbed they begin moving their legs, use their wings and/or legs to become upright, and then begin walking slowly (their wings usually appear droopy when resting or walking). Their feeding behavior appears normal and in rare instances males exhibit sexual calling although it is much less intense than normal males.

distribution of this behavior for both cohorts and individuals? Is supine behavior "reversible" or is it a behavioral marker of impending death?

## Age-specific Morbidity and Mortality Patterns

An event history chart (Carey et al. 1998) showing the age patterns of the supine behavior for each of the 203 males (Fig. 2) reveals a distinct association of individual life span and both the age of onset and the intensity of this behavior. The band depicting supine behavior shows that, in many flies, it begins to occur about 2-3 weeks prior to death; therefore, the period of its occurrence closely follows the cohort survival (lx) schedule. Supine behavior seldom occurred in very young flies (<25 days) but frequently occurred in flies that were over 50 days old - ages at which mortality rates began to increase substantially. The event history chart reveals four general properties of the medfly supine behavior:

1) *persistent* – occurs on subsequent days after onset;
2) *progressive* – intensity increases with age;
3) *predictive* – onset and intensity are strong indicators of impending death; and
4) *universal* – nearly all male medflies exhibit this behavior regardless of their age of death.

Most of the supine behavior began between 10 and 15 days prior to death, with the highest concentrations occurring five to seven days prior to death. Cox propor-

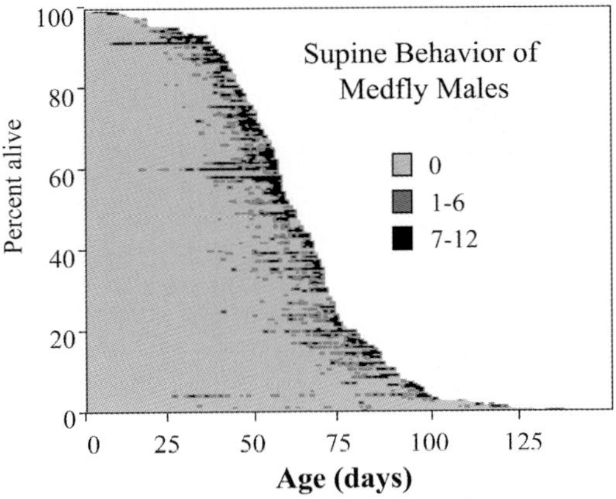


**Fig. 2.** Event history charts for supine behavior in 203 male medflies relative to cohort survival. Each individual is represented by a horizontal line proportional to his life span. Each day an individual that displays supine behavior, it is coded according to the number exhibited: dark gray indicates 1 to 6 supine observations and black indicates 7–12 supine observations.

tional hazards regression models with time-varying predictors were fitted to the data to test for the significance of both onset (pre-supine –to supine) and level of supine behavior with respect to mortality (hazard) rate. The onset of the supine behavior is a highly significant predictor of mortality ($P < 0.0001$) and increases mortality risk considerably more than the level of supine behavior. The model showed that a fly's mortality risk increased by nearly 40-fold once it began exhibiting supine behavior. The level of supine behavior is also a significant predictor of mortality and, for every increase in supine level by 1.0, the hazard rate increases by 26.3%. Fitting a model that has both the onset and level of supine behavior as predictors indicates that both are highly significant, with mortality risk ratios of 17.59 and 1.18 for onset and level of supine behavior, respectively.

## Hazard Rates

Three hazard rates derived from the medfly data are presented in Figure 3, including:

1) *To supine.* This is the hazard rate for the transition from the pre-supine to the supine state, defined as the first observation of any supine behavior. Note the near-linear or Gompertz-like increase in hazard with age, which reveals the ever-increasing likelihood that a fly will experience supine as it ages.
2) *Supine – to death.* This is the supine age-specific death rate, where supine age refers to the number of days since a fly first exhibited supine behavior. This hazard function increases from an initial level of 0.04 at the time of the first supine behavior to a peak of nearly 0.08 at 20 days (supine age). This hazard rate then gradually decreases for the next 30 days to around 0.05 at 50 days (supine

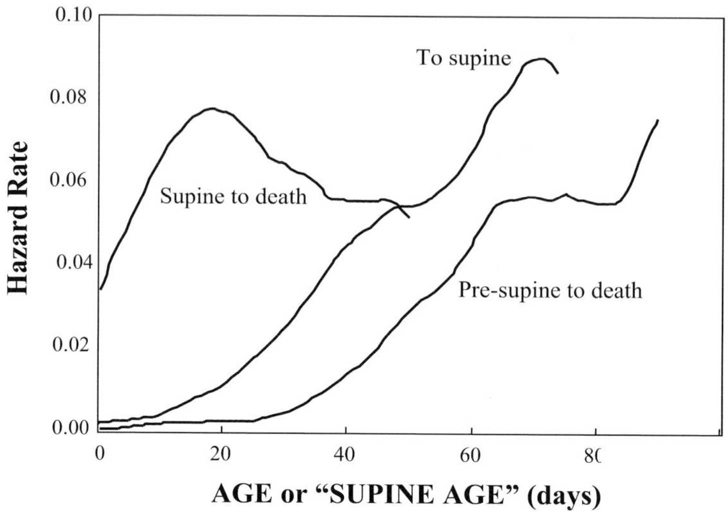


**Fig. 3.** Hazard rates for three transitions observed in male medflies including 'to supine', 'supine-to-death', and 'pre-supine-to-death' (see text).

age). Because the death rate of a pre-supine fly is substantially lower than the death rate of a supine fly, the rate at which pre-supine flies enter the supine state will determine the age pattern of death in the cohort; for a fly to be in the supine state is to be in the state of impending death.

3) *Birth – to death.* This hazard rate is the background age-specific death rate for pre-supine flies. The curve corresponding to this rate that is shown in Figure 3 reveals the reduced probability of a fly dying in the pre-supine state relative to dying in the supine state or of transitioning to the supine condition. In other words, the longer a pre-supine fly can remain in this state rather than transition to supine with higher hazard rates of death, the longer it will live. Note that the death rate of a pre-supine fly does not equal the death rate of a fly newly transitioned into the supine state (i.e., first day in supine state) until it is two months old.

## Life Expectancy Disaggregated by Supine Status

The impact on mortality risk of the onset of supine behavior is illustrated in Figure 4, which shows the remaining life expectancy at each age for all flies (middle curve) as well as flies disaggregated according to whether they had exhibited supine behavior (lower curve) or not (upper curve). Three aspects of this figure merit special comment. First, striking differences occurred in the remaining life of young flies (<20 days) that had not exhibited supine behavior and young flies that were exhibiting supine behavior: the former had over 50-60 days of life remaining (non-supine) but the latter had only 20 days or less left (supine). Sec-

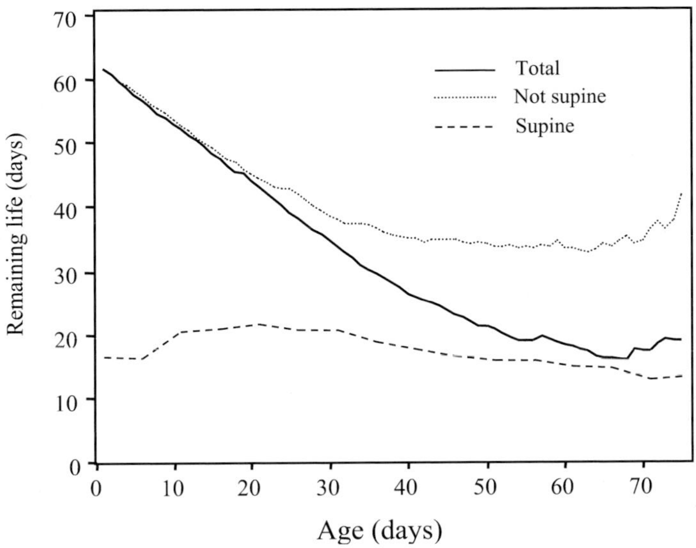


**Fig. 4.** Schedules of remaining life expectancy (days) for male medflies for the cohort as a whole (center line) as well for males both prior to (top line) and after (bottom line) the onset of supine behavior.

ond, the remaining life expectancy of a non-supine fly between 25 and 70 days of age remained constant at about 35 life-days. However, once it entered the supine state, its life expectancy immediately dropped by 20 days to approximately 15 days. Third, the remaining life of flies that initiated the supine behavior was also remarkably constant, ranging from slightly over 20 days for flies that were 10 to 30 days old to around 16-18 days for very young flies and flies older than 30 days.

## "Active" and Total Life Expectancies

We used the age at which a male medfly first exhibited supine behavior to demarcate the end of the "active" period of a fly's life to construct a cohort schedule of "active life" (Katz et al. 1983; Manton and Land 2000). This schedule, combined with the conventional survival ($l_x$) schedule, was used to estimate the age distribution and prevalence of inactive life by taking the difference at each age between the inactive and total life schedules (Fig. 5). Total and active life expectancies were computed as 61.7 and 45.6 days, respectively (Carey 2001) and thus the average male experienced 16.1 days or 26.1% of its 61.7-day lifetime partially in the supine state. The distribution of inactive life for the cohort varied with age, with the greatest prevalence occurring between 30 and 50 days and the least occurring at the younger and older ages. This measure of inactive life provides information about the dimensions of health and morbidity for a fly, other than death, that can be used as a model system for actuarial analysis as a health-status measure.

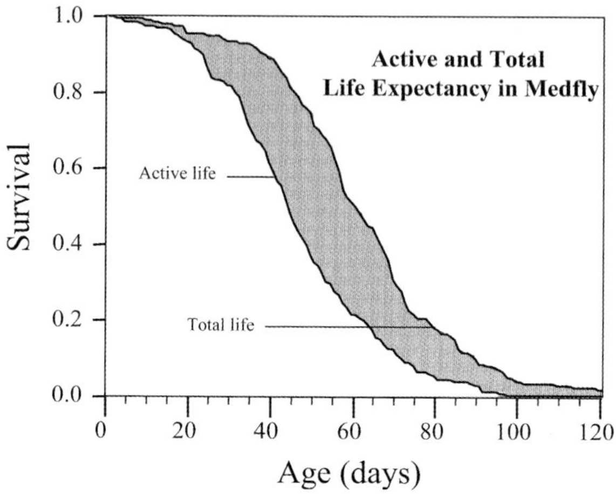


**Fig. 5.** Schedules of active life and total survival for the male medfly cohort. The age at which active life for an individual ended was defined as the age at which supine behavior was first observed. Inactive life was thus defined as all life-days beyond this onset age. This is a schematic example of how the discovery of disablement classification in the medfly can be used to study dynamics of disablement, morbidity and mortality. Nearly all flies become disabled (exhibit supine behavior) prior to death: the average fly spends nearly a quarter of its life in the unhealthy state and never returns to the healthy state. Once a fly is classified as 'unhealthy' (first supine), it has approximately two weeks more of life (Papadopoulos et al. 2002).

## Effects of Changes in Hazard Rates

The morbidity (supine) and mortality hazard rates computed from the medfly data provide useful baselines for use in modeling the impact of changes in these rates on active and total life expectancies and the prevalence of cohort supine behavior. The four patterns of change in morbidity-mortality relationships (Verbrugge and Jette 1994) for each of the hazard rates are presented in Figure 6 and include the following:

**Case #1.** Rising morbidity (supine hazard) and declining mortality. Both total and active life expectancies increase as does the number of fly-days in the supine state because greater numbers of flies survive to the ages at which the "to supine" hazard rates are highest and flies that enter the supine state live longer due to the reduced mortality. Analogous situations for human diseases include diabetes, diseases of the heart, arteriosclerosis, and nephritis.

**Case #2.** Rising morbidity and mortality. In the case shown in Figure 1b, total life expectancy was increased but active life expectancy was decreased, resulting in an increase in the prevalence of morbidity (supine). This is because flies enter the morbid (supine) state at younger ages but the rate of entry into the supine state is not offset by a concomitant increase in mortality. For this case the prevalence of morbidity is conditional on the improvement in morbidity relative to improvement in mortality. Examples of diseases in humans in which both incidence and

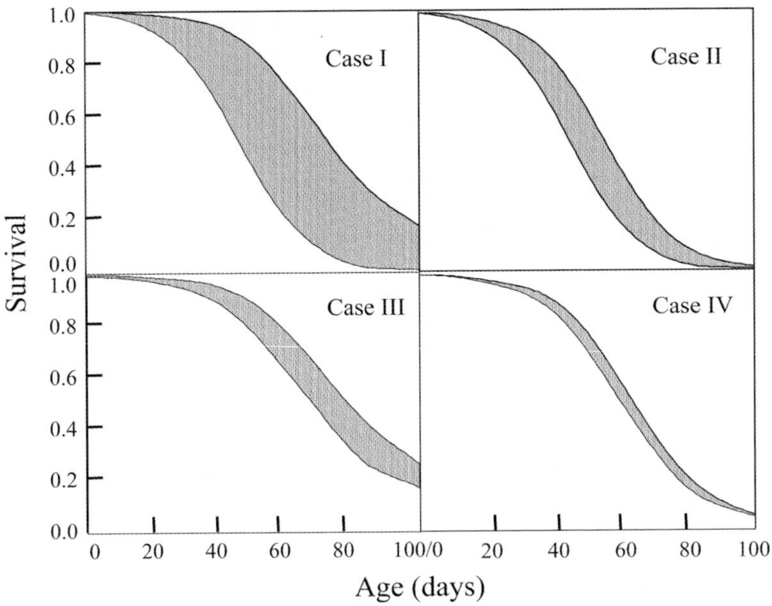


**Fig. 6.** Composite of four scenarios in morbidity and mortality with total and active life expectancies and prevalence of morbidity listed for each case in this respective order. Case I: 65.3, 41.7, and 23.6 days, respectively; Case II: 50.0, 40.6, and 9.4 days, respectively; Case III: 69.3, 61.2, and 8.1 days, respectively; Case IV: 57.6, 54.3, and 3.3 days, respectively.

mortality are increasingly malignant neoplasms, bronchitis, emphysema, and cirrhosis of the liver for individuals aged 45 to 64.

**Case #3.** Declining morbidity and mortality. In this case both active and total life expectancies will increase. Examples of diseases in humans in which both incidence and mortality are decreasing include hernias in men older than 65 and nephrosis for individuals aged 45 to 64.

**Case #4.** Declining morbidity but rising mortality. The prevalence of morbidity will decrease in this case because many flies die prior to the onset of morbidity and those that transition to the morbid (supine) state die more quickly. An example of a disease in humans in which the incidence is decreasing but mortality is increasing is cirrhosis of the liver for individuals aged 65 and older.

Modeling these four hypothetical cases of changes in morbidity and mortality is important for at least three reasons:

1) the process fosters a deeper understanding of the underlying demographic trade-offs necessary to generate different levels of life expectancy and morbidity prevalence;
2) the outcome provides a useful frame-of-reference for comparing the outcome of future experiments in which changes in morbidity and mortality are induced through environmental manipulations; and

3) the implicit assumption for the model is that morbidity and mortality are quasi-independent, that there is a dynamic equilibrium in the relationship between morbidity and mortality as life expectancy changes (Manton 1982).

This basic relationship suggests that, if incidence is unchanged, mortality reductions leading to increases in life expectancy can only occur by increasing the duration of the disease and, consequently, its prevalence. However, as Manton noted, for chronic diseases it is useful to consider the way in which duration is increased:

1) by eliminating lethal sequelae such as pneumonia and not affecting the basic rate of progression of the disease process; and
2) by changing the rate of progression of the primary disease process (i.e., reducing disease severity).

In the Morbidity Compression model, the concept of equilibrium is rejected by arguing that mortality and morbidity are at least partly independent. Equilibrium as a demographic concept is important in human demography because it has serious policy implications: mortality reductions are directly linked with the long-term management of chronic diseases that, in turn, are components of primary health services that are likely to increase greatly (Manton 1982). Concerns about the validity of the assumptions underlying the Morbidity Compression model bring to the surface the inherent problems with hypothesis testing based on the results of clinical research: it is not possible to conduct manipulative frailty experiments on humans. These experiments can only be done with animal models.

## Towards a general research framework

### Importance of Animal Models

Research on impairment using model systems (non-human animals) in both the laboratory and the wild are important because

1) the results of comparative studies will identify common threads in the disablement process across species as well as at different biological levels (molecular, physiological, whole-organism);
2) studies may shed new and important light on the identification of preclinical signals of disablement in non-human species and identify valid methods to determine if these same signals occur in humans and are related to aging;
3) investigations will encourage development of novel concepts and approaches for understanding fundamental aspects of the disablement process rather than characteristics that are idiosyncratic to humans;
4) aging research on the determinants of endpoints other than death (e.g., onset of impairment, disabling or chronic conditions) will provide context and perspectives on mechanisms underlying aging as well as deeper insights into the manifestations of aging including co-morbidity and the sequence of onset, duration of conditions, and the relationship to mortality; and

5) the focus on general properties will foster the creation of a set of general principles of disablement that are as relevant to insects and other invertebrates as they are to humans and other vertebrates and, in turn, encourage the creation of a new research paradigm for manipulating environmental conditions and for hypothesis testing.

This last point is important because of bioethical issues that arise in manipulative research on human subjects as well as the time and cost constraints of longitudinal studies.

## Ecology of Impairment

The vast majority of animals in the wild live on the razor's edge of physical and cognitive fitness. The onset of any physical impairment that would be a nuisance in a protected environment (laboratory or zoo) is virtually a death sentence in the wild. Any animal that no longer possesses the speed, strength and agility to forage for food to escape danger is at great risk in nature; arthritic lions that have difficulty quelling and killing large prey; wildebeests exhibiting even the slightest limp that are quickly targeted by sharp-eyed predators. Indeed, locomotor movement is one of the defining characteristics of animals (Biewener 2003), whether the animal is single-celled or has appendages. The specific mechanisms of movement across species are extraordinarily diverse: darting, (hummingbirds), soaring (petrels) and flapping (songbirds) flight in various bird species; lumbering (elephants), prancing (antelope), scurrying (lizards), racing (cheetahs) and running (cockroaches) gaits in terrestrial animals; swimming (otters), paddling (ducks), diving (seals) and flipper-propelled (whales) motion in aquatic animals. Despite the diversity of mechanisms and types of movement, there are a relatively small number of common principles and biological components that underlie these mechanisms, regardless of the medium through which the animals move. It follows that there will be a small number of principles that underlie the loss of function and the acquisition of impairments through physiological, morphological and/or neurological degeneration with age.

## Morbidity Compression in Biodemographic Context

A useful frame of reference for developing a research program in disablement processes in particular is the well-known Compression of Morbidity hypothesis, which was first introduced in 1980 (Fries 1980) and has become the dominant paradigm underlying health improvement programs and policies directed at more successful aging (Fries 1983; Kannisto 2000) Most morbidity results from chronic processes and is concentrated in the years prior to death. The goal is the compression of morbidity between its time of onset (around 55 years) and the age of death (around 75 years). If mortality decreases predominate, there may be more morbidity in a typical life (so-called "failure of success") if the age of onset of chronic disease does not change. However, if the age of onset of chronic disease is increased, then (according to the model) morbidity is compressed, the period of adult vigor is prolonged, life quality is improved, and the need for medical care and associated costs may be reduced (Fries 2000). One of the central issues of medical discoveries of the future is whether they may add health or add illness to the average life. If morbidity is compressed by a new advance, then the advantage is clear; however, if the process of dying is prolonged, then major ethical issues arise (Fries 2000).

### Biodemography of Disability Processes: Generalizing Frailty Concepts

The *International Classification of Functioning, Disability and Health*, known as ICF (WHO 2001), provides a unified and standard language and framework for the description of health and health-related states. It defines components of well-being and domains including 1) body functions and structures and 2) activities and participation. "Functioning" is an umbrella term encompassing all body functions, activities and participation; "disability" serves as an umbrella term for impairments, activity limitations or participation restrictions. "Pathology" refers to biochemical and physiological abnormalities that are detected and medically labeled as disease, injury or developmental condition. "Impairments" are dysfunctions and significant structural abnormalities in specific body systems. They involve the loss or limitation of physical, mental or sensory function on a long term or permanent basis. "Functional limitations" are restrictions on performing fundamental physical and mental actions used in daily life by one's age/sex group. They indicate overall abilities of body and mind to do purposeful work (or make a living in the wild). "Disability" is experienced difficulty doing activities in any domain of life (humans or animals) due to a health or physical problem. Two features of disability are important. First, chronic conditions can affect any activity domain, which, for humans, can include personal care, household management, or employment. For non-human species, this activity domain includes grooming and other hygienic behaviors, food and mate foraging and, for social species, social communication as well as establishment and maintenance of social relationships. Second, the basic feature of disability is difficulty in doing activities in one's regular milieu. Thus visual impairment (short-sightedness) does not become a (very minor) disability until reading is required. The injured leg in a zoo animal does not become a major disability unless the animal is released into the wild. The ICF framework can be used as a preliminary model for disablement studies on non-human species, examples of which are given in Table 1.

## Conclusions

Although the importance of understanding how the behaviors of individuals change with age has long been recognized in honeybees (Frisch 1953) and other social insects (Bourke and Franks 1995; Choe and Crespi 1997) in the context of age polyethism (Seeley 1995; Wilson 1971), the study in which supine behavior in

**Table 1.** Disablement concepts with examples for humans and for the different model systems (possible scenarios).

| Species | Scenario |
|---|---|
| *Humans (Example 1)* | A woman age 74 with osteoarthritis in both hands (pathology) has weak grip and restricted finger flexion (impairments). This causes difficulty in grasping and rotating fixed objects (functional limitations), and she has trouble opening jars or doors (disability). She purchases kitchen devices and special door handles (interventions) to overcome the difficulty (Verbrugge and Jette 1994). |
| *Humans (Example 2)* | A woman age 90 has no specific diagnoses (pathology), but her sight, hearing, and senses of taste and smell have diminished significantly in recent years and she is forgetful and feels confused (impairments). Gradually she stops socializing (disability) and becomes deeply depressed (quality-of-life outcome). She spends most of the time tearful and seated (functional limitations; feedback effects from disability). Her physical frailty steadily increases (impairment; feedback effect from functional limitation). One night she dies while sleeping (Verbrugge and Jette 1994). |
| *Nematodes* | A 23-day-old, post-reproductive (pathology) nematode rarely moves (impairment) because it has released all of its eggs and thus has no need to forage for the food (bacteria) required to produce more eggs. With no motivation for feeding (disability) but because it is a long-lived DAF-2 mutant, it lives for another month in a quasi-suspended state before it eventually wastes away and dies at 53 days. |
| *Medflies* | A 68-day-old medfly female has a damaged wing (pathology) and thus has difficulty flying (impairment). This causes difficulty in reaching the food located in a small container suspended from the cage top (functional limitation) and thus increases the risk of becoming weak or of dying due to inability to reach food (disability). Thus food is placed on the cage floor within easy reach (intervention). |
| *Honeybee* | A 25-day-old worker bee is weakened due to a parasite infection (pathology) and thus suffers from restricted mobility (impairment), including within-hive movement needed for brood care and pollen foraging outside the colony (functional limitation). This increases the risk of death due to its rejection by other workers within the hive and because of its reduced ability to navigate and avoid predation while foraging (Rueppell et al. 2004). |
| *Mouse* | A 17-month-old female mouse that, when younger, regularly used the treadmill, now suffers from progressive renal failure (pathology). She is listless and weak (impairment) and thus seldom feeds or uses the treadmill (disability). She spends much time curled up in a corner of the cage chewing on her tail (feedback from impairment) until she eventually dies. |
| *Macaque* | A 22-year-old male macaque is injured (pathology) in a fight with a younger male and suffers partial paralysis in one arm (impairment). This causes difficulty in both climbing and self-defense (functional limitation), which, in turn, reduces his social status, heightens stress levels and reduces access to food (disability). He spends most of the time in isolation (functional limitations; feedback effects from disability), receives little grooming and shows loss of condition (quality-of-life outcome). One day, he is attacked at feeding time by other males and dies of his injuries. |

medflies was first discovered appears to be the first to systematically record and analyze data on the age patterns of behavior from birth to death for a non-social insect. Indeed, we could not find any other relatively large-scale study in which age-specific behavior was recorded over the lifetime of individuals. Not only was a new (supine) behavior discovered in the medfly investigation but the frequency of occurrence of supine was found to be a biomarker of aging and a predictor of impending death. Thus the study opens up new possibilities for experimental studies of frailty in model systems and with this, the opportunity to both re-visit and extend existing paradigms in disability studies and the demography of frailty. In particular, the hypothesis that morbidity and mortality are quasi or partially independent needs to be rigorously tested in model systems. We believe that it will not be possible to develop principles that are truly basic until experimental methods, animal models, and hypothesis testing are integrated into the existing, clinically based paradigm of frailty and disability studies. And without these basic concepts and principles, research on frailty will lack a coherency and a theoretical foundation that are essential for advancing the field.

## References


Albrecht GL, Seelman, KD, Bury, M (2001) Handbook of disability studies. SAGE Pub., Thousand Oaks, California.

Baker GT, Sprott, RL (1988) Biomarkers of aging. Expl Gerontol 23: 223-239

Biewener AA (2003) Animal locomotion, Oxford University Press, Oxford

Bourke AFG, Franks NR (1995) Social Evolution in Ants. Princeton University Press, Princeton

Carey JR (2001) Insect biodemography Annu Rev Entomol 46: 79-110

Carey JR, Liedo P, Muller HG, Wang JL, Vaupel JW (1998) A simple graphical technique for displaying individual fertility data and cohort survival: case study of 1000 Mediterranean fruit fly females. Func Ecol 12: 359-363

Choe JC, Crespi BJ (1997) Social behavior in insects and arachnids. Cambridge University Press, Cambridge

Fries JF (1980) Aging, natural death, and the compression of morbidity. New Engl J Med 303:130-135

Fries JF (1983) The compression of morbidity. Milbank Mem Fund Quart /Hlth Soc 61: 397-419

Fries J F (2000) Compression of morbidity in the elderly. Vaccine 18: 1584-1589.

Frisch KV (1953) The dancing bees: an account of the life and Senses of the honey bee. Harvest Book, New York

Kannisto V (2000) Measuring the compression of mortality. Demog Res 3: 1-24

Katz S, Branch LG, Branson MH, Papsidero JA, Beck JC, Greer DS (1983) Active life expectancy. New Engl J Med 309: 1218-1224

Lollar DJ, Crews JE (2003) Redefining the role of public health in disability. Annu Rev Pub Hlth 24: 195-208

Manton KG (1982) Changing concepts of morbidity and mortality in the elderly population. Milbank Mem Fund Quart/Hlth Soc 60: 183-244

Manton KG, Land KC (2000) Active life expectancy estimates for the US elderly population: a multidimensional continuous-mixture model of functional change applied to completed cohorts, 1982-1996. Demography 37: 253-265

Manton KG, Gu, X (2001) Changes in the prevalence of chronic disability in the United States black and non black population above age 65 from 1982 to 1999. Proc Natl Acad Sci 98: 6354-6359

Manton KG, Corder L, Stallard E (1997) Chronic disability trends in elderly United States populations: 1982-1994. Proc Natl Acad Sci 94: 2593-2598

Markowska AL, Breckler SJ (1999) Behavioural biomarkers of aging: illustration of a multivariate approach for detecting age-related behavioural changes. J Geron Biol Sci 12: B549-B566

Mehrotra A, Dudley RA, Luft, HS (2002) What's behind the health expenditure trends? Annu Rev Pub Hlth 24: 385-412

Papadopoulos NT, Carey JR, Katsoyannos BI, Kouloussis NA, Müller HG, Liu X (2002) Supine behaviour predicts time-to-death in male Mediterranean fruit flies Proc Roy Soc London: Biol Sci 269: 1633-1637

Papadopoulos NT, Katsoyannos BI, Kouloussis NA, Carey JR, Müller HG, Zhang Y (2004) High sexual calling rates predict extended life span in male Mediterranean fruit flies. Oecologia 138: 127-134

Rueppell O, Amdam GV, Page RE Jr, Carey JR (2004) From genes to societies. Science Aging Knowledge Environment 5: pe5

Seeley TD (1995) The wisdom of the hive: The social physiology of honey bee colonies. Harvard University Press, London

Singer BH, Manton KG (1998) The effects of health changes on projections of health service needs for the elderly population of the United States. Proc Natl Acad Sci USA: 15618-15622

Verbrugge LM, Jette AM (1994) The disablement process. Soc Sci Med 38: 1-14

WHO (2001) International classification of functioning, disability and health. World Health Organization, Geneva

Wilson EO (1971) The insect societies, The Belknap Press of Harvard University Press, Cambridge, MA

# Social control of aging and frailty in bees

*Gro V. Amdam*[1]

## Summary

Fertility is not inversely correlated with longevity in social insects. This fact seems contrary to the norm in solitary model organisms, where experimental manipulations that result in longer life spans often act on reproductive pathways and reduce fertility. In social insects, however, reproduction is divided between two female phenotypes: the queens that are locked into a continuous oviposition mode, and the workers that express the remaining range of maternal functions, such as preparation of oviposition sites, nest defense, brood care, hygienic behaviors, and foraging. In the social honey bee, workers show a flexible aging pattern as they shift between behaviors that are associated with different aging rates. The behavioral repertoire of a honey bee worker is usually expressed in a sequence, so that tasks associated with rapid senescence follow tasks associated with slow or negligible senescence. However, when prompted by changes in colony demography, bees can respond with behavioral reversions and acquire physiological states associated with slower aging. This plasticity emerges in part through an interplay between a systemic hormone and a gene normally expressed exclusively by reproductive females. The genetic networks that control aging in sterile worker bees may have evolved through decoupling and subsequent remodeling of regulatory architectures that linked senescence and fertility in their solitary predecessor. The aging machinery of honey bees may, therefore, provide new knowledge about the structure, plasticity and evolvability of pathways that shape the course of aging and frailty.

## Introduction

Research on pathways that regulate senescence has identified endocrine signaling cascades that regulate reproduction and longevity (e.g., reviewed by Tatar et al. 2003). Insulin/insulin-like growth factor signaling (IIS) affects adult fecundity and aging in the nematode, *Caenorhabditis elegans*, through separate regulatory events in the larval and adult stages (Dillin et al. 2002). The IIS-pathway is evo-

[1] Department of Entomology, University of California, Davis, 95616 CA, U.S.A., and Department of Animal and Aquacultural Sciences, Norwegian University of Life Sciences, N-1432 Aas, Norway

Carey et al.
Longevity and Frailty

lutionarily conserved, and in the fly, *Drosophila melanogaster*, it affects ovariole number (i.e., ovary size) through activity in the larva (Tu and Tatar 2003); it influences senescence, however, by signaling in the adult fly. This finding suggests that regulatory events that link reproduction and longevity are at least partly sequentially segregated throughout the life cycle of many organisms.

Social insect females can develop into reproductive and non-reproductive forms that are characterized by different morphology, physiology, and behavior. These "castes" may have evolved through developmental segregating and subsequent truncation of stages that, in sum, made up the life cycle of their solitary predecessor (West-Eberhard 1987, 1996; Amdam et al. 2004a). Accordingly, each caste does not proceed through a complete repertoire of female behaviors and functions (Fig. 1). Endocrine, physiological and behavioral events confined to specific life stages may have dissociated through caste segregation (Amdam et al. 2004a). It is, therefore, interesting to note that fertility is not inversely linked to longevity in social insects (Finch 1990), as this pattern might suggest that regulatory actions that associated reproduction with senescence in the pre-social ancestor dissociated during social evolution. A deeper understanding of the regulatory architectures that shape patterns of senescence in social insects may, therefore, be an important contribution to our understanding of aging. This perspective is elucidated in the following paper outlining current knowledge about aging in the social honey bee (*Apis mellifera*).

## Aging and frailty in honey bees

The honey bee has two female castes, the reproductive queens (Fig. 1B) and the functionally sterile workers (Fig. 1C). A honey bee egg can, in principle, develop into both, but differential feeding during the larval stage results in a bifurcation that separate the development trajectories of the two castes. Subsequently, the long-lived queens have large ovaries and are arrested in continuous oviposition mode. They never forage, prepare oviposition sites, defend the nest or feed brood (the developing larvae). Workers, on the other hand, display a flexible aging pattern linked to the remaining range of female functions, including brood care and foraging (Fig. 2); reviewed by Omholt and Amdam 2004; see Winston 1987 for further information on honey bee biology).

Overall, the honey bee shows positive linkage between the rate of senescence and the magnitude of extrinsic mortality (Finch 1990), as predicted by evolutionary theories of aging (e.g., reviewed by Kirkwood and Austad 2000). However, a single honey bee genotype can generate four adult phenotypes characterized by separate aging patterns (Fig. 2A). The queen caste that senesces at negligible rates is one (possible mechanisms reviewed by Finch 1990), while the workers express the remaining three (Omholt and Amdam 2004; see also Fig. 2A): 1) the *diutinus* phenotype, which develops in the absence of brood (Maurizio 1950; Fluri et al. 1977, 1982). It remains highly protected inside the colony, where it thermoregulates the nest at 28–33°C and cares for the queen during periods of unfavorable conditions (e.g., rain and snow). It can live for more than 280 days and is characterized by very high levels of storage protein (an amino acid source for self-

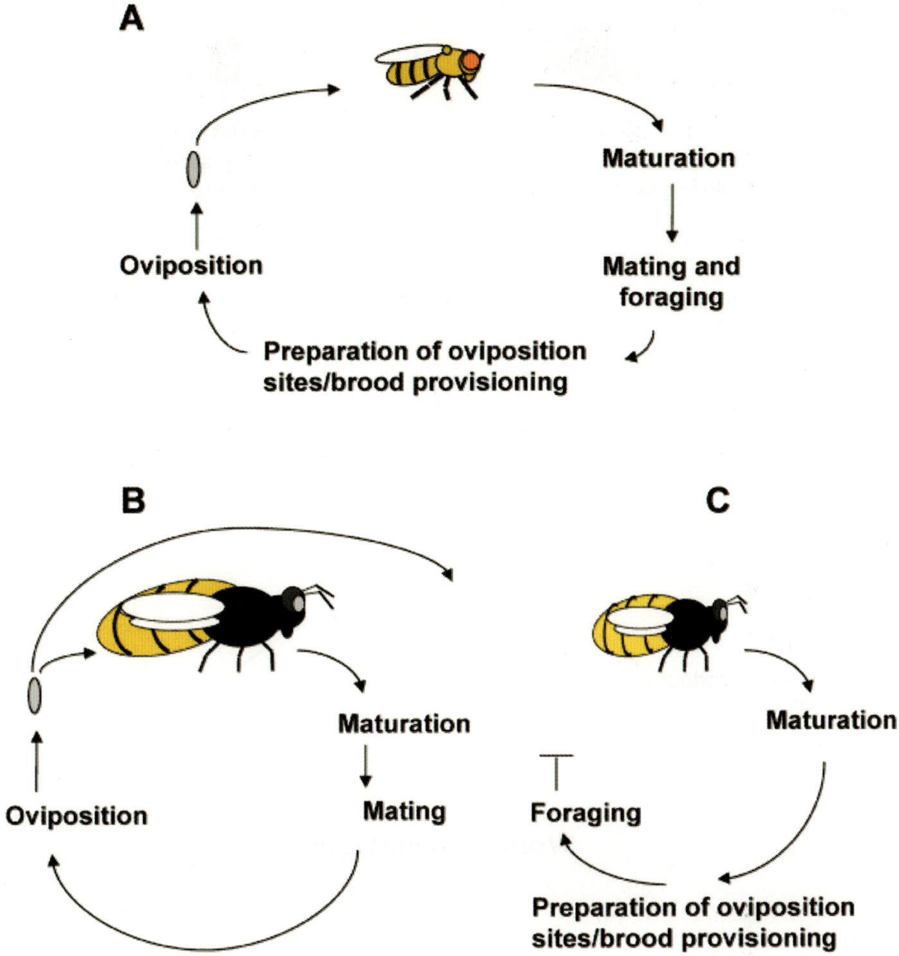


**Fig 1.** Compartmentalization of female functions in social insects. Solitary insect females go through complete cycles of female functions (**A**), whereas social insects show reproductive division of labor (**B,C**). Females are either reproductive queens (**B**) or non-reproductive workers (**C**). Together, the two castes complete a full set of female life stages. Relative to each other, however, they show reciprocal deletions of sequential phases in the life cycle of the solitary insect.

maintenance) and high numbers of functional immune cells (8,000–10,000 per μl hemolymph); 2) the hive bee phenotype, which engages in brood care within the protected nest. It has an upper lifespan of 75–135 days, moderate levels of storage protein, and intermediate numbers of functional immune cells (4,500–8,000 per μl); and 3) the forager phenotype, which performs risky nectar- and pollen-collecting behaviors outside the colony. It can live for 7–14 days, is deprived of storage protein, and has few or no functional immune cells (0–1,000 per μl). The low

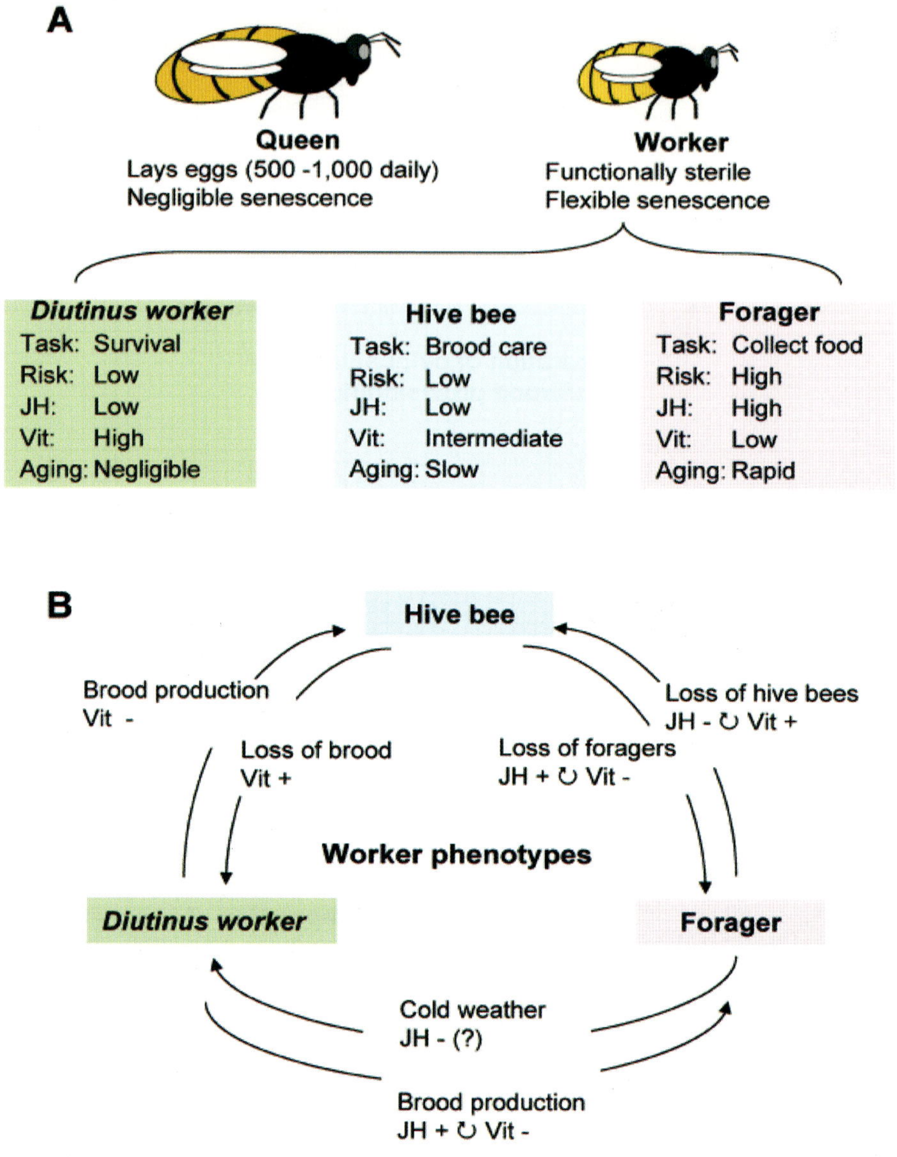


**Fig. 2.** Polyphenisms of aging in honey bees. (**A**) Honey bee queens reside within the highly protected nests and experience negligible mechanical and physiological senescence (Finch 1990). Workers normally do not lay eggs and can develop three adult phenotypes characterized by distinct aging rates. The three forms have distinct behavioral profiles (Task) with associated extrinsic mortality risks (Risk). They also differ in their hemolymph level of the systemic hormone juvenile hormone (JH) and the *vg* gene product vitellogenin (Vit). A worker will switch between phenotypes as a function of the social condition (**B**). Associated shifts in aging rate appear to be driven by interplay between JH and the activity of the *vg* gene. In the specific case of forager reversion to *diutinus* function, a stress-resistant survival stage, low ambient temperatures may also be a factor (see Huang and Robinson 1995 for a discussion).

immunocyte count appears to result from extensive pycnasis (cell death) (Amdam et al. 2004b).

Information about associated frailty patterns is limited, but hive bees senesce after 30–75 days as their ability to nurse brood declines (Haydak 1963; Eischen et al. 1984). The foragers' performance appears to go down after as few as five days (Tofilski 2000), whereas *diutinus* workers can shift to efficient nursing and foraging when as old as 280 days (Sakagami and Fukuda 1968; Terada et al. 1975). Furthermore, a recent study demonstrates that *diutinus* workers, hive bees, and foragers differ in their resistance to the oxidative-damage agent, paraquat (Seehuus et al., manuscript in preparation). Oxidative-stress resistance is an important biomarker of aging, and the results of Seehuus et al. (in preparation) indicate that resistance to stress is not a function of chronological age in bees: 30-day-old foragers were frailer than 30-day-old hive bees, whereas the lowest levels of frailty were found in *diutinus* workers that were older than 200 days. This finding suggests that individual bees show task-related patterns of physiological frailty that at least partly correspond to the extrinsic mortality risk associated with each activity. However, bees in the same cohort do not shift between tasks at the same age, and similarly aged bees can sometimes develop into both foragers and *diutinus* workers (Huang and Robinson 1995). This finding may indicate that mortality in honey bees is particularly heterogeneous (Vaupel et al. 1979).

The honey bee worker phenotypes are usually expressed in a sequence, so that the tasks associated with rapid senescence (foraging) follow tasks associated with slow (hive bee duties) or negligible senescence (*diutinus* function). Furthermore, the bees respond to subtle changes in colony demography by adjusting their progression through this succession of tasks. A moderate increase in forager mortality, therefore, results in a moderate increase in the number of bees that shifts from nursing to foraging (Huang and Robinson 1996). More dramatic demographic changes, however, can trigger shifts from phenotypes characterized by rapid aging to states associated with slower aging (Fig. 2B). Specifically, extensive removal of hive bees causes bees to stop foraging and to develop physiological and behavioral features associated with brood care (Huang and Robinson 1996; for further information, see Figure 2B). The longevity patterns of bees are, thus, functions of the social condition, which implies that honey bee aging is largely under social control (Omholt and Amdam 2004).

## Polyphenisms of honey bee aging

The aging pattern of bees may be described as "polyphenic" (Omholt et al, manuscript in preparation), which signifies a genome's ability to produce two or more alternative phenotypes in response to environmental stimuli. Polyphenisms of aging are also found in *C. elegans*, which has a specialized third larval stage, *dauer*, adapted for survival under unfavorable conditions (Riddle 1977; Riddle et al.; 1981). *Dauer* formation, in which animals undergo a metabolic shift to a long-lived, stress-resistant dispersal form, is induced by high population densities and low amounts of food (reviewed by Vanfleteren and Braeckman 1999). *Drosophila* that over-winter as adults in reproductive diapause also age at negligible rates and are stress-resistant (Tatar et al. 2001). Phenotypic plasticity in aging rates is, therefore, a common phenomenon. The number of aging polyphenisms appears to be particularly high in the honey bee, however. The flexibility that emerges from the capacity of workers to make bidirectional shifts between phenotypes also seems to be unsurpassed by conventional model organisms used in aging research.

## Regulation of honey bee longevity

The honey bee *vg* gene codes for the conserved yolk precursor vitellogenin that, as a rule, is synthesized exclusively by oviparous females prior to egg formation (see Amdam and Omholt 2002 for a review). The *vg* gene is, however, also expressed at high levels in hive bees and *diutinus* workers, where it appears to have evolved new functions. The hive bees use the zinc-carrying glyco-lipoprotein product to feed larvae (Amdam et al. 2003a); therefore, vitellogenin accumulates in the *diutinus* workers that live in absence of brood (Omholt and Amdam 2004). It has been suggested that workers can use vitellogenin as a storage protein for self-maintenance, and that the hemolymph (blood) concentrations in hive bees (~30 μg/ul) and *diutinus* workers (~100 μg/ul) therefore partly reflect the relative longevity potential of the two groups (Amdam et al. 2004c). Furthermore, down-regulation of *vg* activity by RNA interference demonstrates that task-associated patterns of frailly to paraquat are at least partly linked to the relative vitellogenin level in the workers (Seehuus et al., manuscript in preparation). Seehuus et al. also present molecular evidence indicating that vitellogenin has an antioxidant function.

A link between the systemic hormone juvenile hormone (JH), the zinc-binding function of vitellogenin and the number of functional hemocytes has also been discovered in bees. *Diutinus* workers and hive bees have low JH levels, but the JH titer increases when bees start foraging. The high JH level shuts down *vg* activity (Pinto et al. 2000), which causes the hemolymph zinc level to drop from 10–25 ppm to 0–4 ppm (Amdam et al. 2004b). Normal immunocyte function in insects appears to require at least 7 ppm of zinc, and cultures of honey bee hemocytes incubated at 0–4 ppm zinc show significant decline relative to cultures kept at 25 ppm (Amdam et al. 2004b). The negative effect of JH on the *vg* gene may, therefore, be partially responsible for the low number of functional immune cells in foragers (reviewed by Omholt and Amdam 2004). Note that JH does not affect *vg* gene expression in adult queens, which have vitellogenin titers in the range of *diutinus* workers (Rutz and Lüscher 1974; Fluri et al. 1981). In bees, JH appears to have lost gonotropic functions that are common in solitary insect females (Hartfelder 2000). The same phenomenon has been confirmed for ecdysone (Hartfelder et al. 2002), which is another systemic hormone that is involved in the aging regulation of *Drosophila* (reviewed by Tatar et al. 2003 see also Fig. 3A).

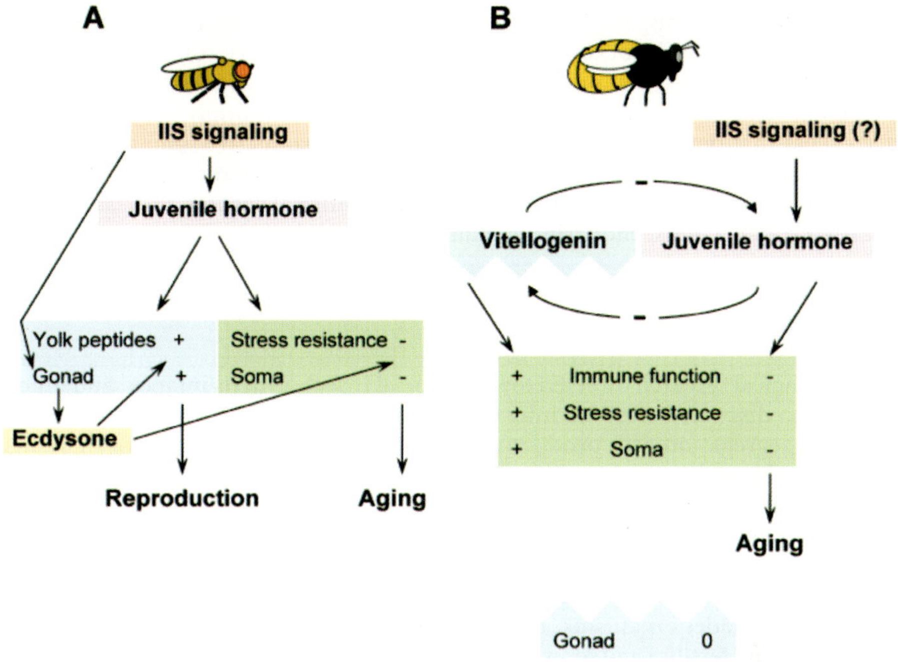


**Fig. 3.** Outline of regulatory circuits of aging in fly and bee. Direct or indirect insulin signaling (IIS) triggers JH and ecdysone production in *Drosophila* (**A**), which co-regulates yolk peptide expression (positive) and gonad development (positive) in antagonism with somatic maintenance (negative). In the honey bee worker (**B**), the *vg* gene product, vitellogenin, has been integrated in the somatic maintenance machinery and has a positive effect on life span. Vitellogenin is a yolk protein that has immunological, antioxidant and amino acid storage functions. It feeds back on the JH control system and can suppress JH synthesis. JH's action on *vg* is inverted relative to the fly, so high levels suppress yolk protein production. Through these regulatory relationships, JH and the *vg* gene are clocked in a regulatory feedback loop. The directional effect of JH on somatic maintenance is conserved between fly and bee (negative). JH and ecdysone have dissociated from gonotropic roles in both workers and queens, however, and the co-regulatory link to the gonad has, therefore, been decoupled. No putative roles of ecdysone in honey bee aging are currently known.

## Regulatory remodeling of aging

JH is part of the IIS pathway in *Drosophila* (e.g., Tatar et al. 2003), where it co-regulates yolk peptide expression and somatic maintenance antagonistically (Fig. 3A). Similarly, the vitellogenin genes *vit-2* and *vit-5* are down-stream of the IIS receptor *daf-2* in *C. elegans*, and reduction of their activities lengthens life span (Murphy et al. 2003). In the bee worker, however, *vg* expression has a positive effect on stress resistance and longevity, and the regulatory action of JH on the *vg* gene is inverted so that high JH levels suppress vitellogenin synthesis (Pinto et al. 2000). It was recently shown that the *vg* gene also feeds back on the hormonal control system (Guidugli et al. manuscript in preparation), and may suppress JH to produce long-lived worker bees (Fig. 3B). This regulatory role of vitellogenin has never before been demonstrated, although the coding gene is conserved over oviparous taxa (Mann et al. 1999). These findings may imply that evolutionary events that detached JH and ecclysone from reproductive functions in bees opened for remodeling of the regulatory circuits of aging and reproduction. The resulting dynamics, therefore diverge from conventional wisdom on associations between yolk proteins, endocrine signaling and aging.

## Perspectives

Gerontological research directed towards social insects is in its infancy, and much remains to discover before we fully understand the mechanics of caste evolution and how segregation of reproductive castes may have affect regulatory circuits that control longevity and fertility. However, our current understanding of honey bee aging indicates that further dissections of the regulatory machineries that control senescence in this social insect may provide new knowledge about the pathways that shape the course of aging and frailty. Several findings suggest that elements of pathways responsible for aging diverge between the social honey bee and solitary model organisms. First, loss of JH and ecdysone functions and the pairing of high fertility and long life span in queens might point to developmental decoupling of circuits that normally produce negative associations between fertility and longevity. Second, the inverse regulatory relationship between JH and the *vg* gene, the integration of the protein product vitellogenin in the somatic maintenance machinery, and the control-action of *vg* on the endocrine system of workers suggest that honey bees have evolved novelties in their regulatory circuits of aging. The directional effect of JH on somatic maintenance (negative) is conserved in workers, however. This association may imply that other elements of IIS signaling are conserved as well.

Aging is a universal process in living organisms, but information about interspecific variability in structure, plasticity, and evolvability of aging regulation is still limited. It is therefore encouraging to note that several functional genomic tools have been established for bees (Robinson et al. 2000; Beye et al. 2002; Amdam et al. 2003b), and the honey bee genome is almost completely sequenced (see http://hgsc.bcm.tmc.edu/index.html ).

## Acknowledgment

Funding was provided by the Norwegian Research Council, project no. 157851/432, NIA PO1 AG 22500, and Fondation IPSEN.

## References

Amdam GV, Omholt SW (2002) The regulatory anatomy of honeybee lifespan. J Theor Biol 216: 209–228

Amdam GV, Norberg K, Hagen A, Omholt SW (2003a) Social exploitation of vitellogenin. Proc Natl Acad Sci USA 100: 1799–1802

Amdam GV, Simões ZLP, Guidugli KR, Norberg K, Omholt SW (2003b) Disruption of vitellogenin gene function in adult honeybees by intra-abdominal injection of double-stranded RNA. BMC Biotechnol 3: 1–8

Amdam GV, Norberg K, Fondrk MK, Page RE (2004a) Reproductive ground plan may mediate colony-level selection effects on individual foraging behavior in honey bees. Proc Natl Acad Sci USA 101: 11350–11355

Amdam GV, Simões ZLP, Hagen A, Norberg K, Schrøder K, Mikkelsen Ø, Kirkwood TBL, Omholt SW (2004b) Hormonal control of the yolk precursor vitellogenin regulates immune function and longevity in honeybees. Exp Gerontol 39: 767–773

Amdam GV, Hartfelder K, Norberg K, Hagen A, Omholt SW (2004c) Altered physiology in worker honey bees (Hymenoptera: Apidae) infested by the mite *Varroa destructor* (Acari: Varroidae): a factor in colony loss during over-wintering? J Econ Entomol 97: 741–747

Beye M, Hartel S, Hagen A, Hasselmann M, Omholt SW (2002) Specific developmental gene silencing in the honey bee using a homeobox motif. Insect Mol Biol 11: 527–532

Dillin A, Crawford DK, Kenyon C (2002) Timing requirements for insulin/IGF-1 signaling in C. elegans. Science 298: 830–834

Eischen FA, Rothenbuhler WC, Kulincevic JM (1984) Some effects of nursing on nurse bees. J Apic Re. 23: 90–93

Finch CE (1990) Longevity, senescence and the genome. Chicago: University of Chicago Press

Fluri P, Wille H, Gerig L, Lüscher M (1977) Juvenile hormone, vitellogenin and haemocyte composition in winter worker honeybees (Apis mellifera). Experientia 33: 1240–1241

Fluri P, Sabatini AG, Vecchi MA, Wille H (1981) Blood juvenile hormone, protein and vitellogenin titres in laying and non-laying queen honeybees. J Apic Res 20: 221–225

Fluri P, Lüscher M, Wille H, Gerig L (1982) Changes in weight of the pharyngeal gland and haemolymph titres of juvenile hormone, protein and vitellogenin in worker honey bees. J Insect Physiol 28: 61–68

Hartfelder K (2000) Insect juvenile hormone: from "status quo" to high society. Braz J Med Biol Res 33: 157–177

Hartfelder K, Bitondi MMG, Santana WC, Simões ZLP (2002) Ecdysteroid titer and reproduction in queens and workers of the honey bee and of a stingless bee: loss of ecdysteroid function at increasing levels of sociality? Insect Biochem Molec Biol 32: 211–216

Haydak MH (1963) Age of nurse bees and brood rearing. Minnesota Agric Exp Station, Scientific J. Series No. 5122: 101–103

Huang Z-Y, Robinson GE (1995) Seasonal changes in juvenile hormone titers and rates of biosynthesis in honey bees. J Comp Physiol B 165: 18–28

Huang Z-Y, Robinson GE (1996) Regulation of honey bee division of labor by colony age demography. Behav Ecol Sociobiol 39: 147–158

Kirkwood TBL, Austad SN (2000) Why do we age? Nature 408: 233–237

Mann CJ, Anderson TA, Read J, Chester SA, Harrison GB, Köchl S, Ritchie PJ, Bradbury P, Hussain FS, Amey J, Vanloo B, Rosseneu M, Infante R, Hancock JM, Levitt DG, Banaszak LJ, Scott J, Shoulders CC (1999) The structure of vitellogenin provides a molecular model for the assembly and secretion of atherogenic lipoproteins. J Molec Biol 285: 391–408

Maurizio A (1950) The influence of pollen feeding and brood rearing on the length of life and physiological condition of the honeybee preliminary report. Bee World 31: 9–12

Murphy CT, McCarroll SA, Bargmann CI, Fraser A, Kamath RS, Ahringer J, Li H, Kenyon C (2003) Genes that act downstream of DAF-16 to influence the lifespan of Caenorhabditis elegans. Nature 424: 277–284

Omholt SW, Amdam GV (2004) Epigenic regulation of aging in honeybee workers. Sci Aging Knowl Environ 26: pe28
Pinto LZ, Bitondi MMG, Simões ZLP (2000) Inhibition of vitellogenin synthesis in Apis mellifera workers by a juvenile hormone analogue, pyriproxyfen. Insect Physiol 46: 153–160
Riddle DL (1977) Genetic pathway for dauer larva formation in nematode, Caenorhabditis-elegans. Genetics 86: S51–S52
Riddle DL, Swanson MM, Albert PS (1981) Interacting genes in nematode dauer larva formation. Nature 290: 668–671
Robinson KO, Fergusson HJ, Cobey S, Vaessin H, Smith BH (2000) Sperm-mediated transformation of the honey bee, Apis mellifera. Insect Molec Biol 9: 625–634
Rutz W, Lüscher M (1974) The occurrence of vitellogenin in workers and queens of Apis mellifica and the possibility of its transmission to the queen. J Insect Physiol 20: 897–909
Sakagami SF, Fukuda H (1968) Life tables for worker honeybees. Res Popul Ecol 10: 127–139
Tatar M, Chien SA, Priest NK (2001) Negligible senescence during reproductive dormancy in Drosophila melanogaster. Am Nature 158: 248–258
Tatar M, Bartke A, Antebi A (2003) The endocrine regulation of aging by insulin-like signals. Science 299: 1346–1350
Terada Y, Garofalo CA, Sakagami SF (1975) Age-survival curves for workers of two eusocial bees (Apis mellifera and Plebeia droryana) in a subtropical climate, with notes on worker polyethism in P. droryana. J Apic Res 14: 161–170
Tofilski A (2000) Senescence and learning in honeybee (Apis mellifera) workers. Acta Neurobiol Exp 60: 35–39
Tu MP, Tatar M (2003) Juvenile diet restriction and the aging and reproduction of adult Drosophila melanogaster. Aging Cell 2: 327–333
Vanfleteren JR, Braeckman BP (1999) Mechanisms of life span determination in Caenorhabditis elegans. Neurobiol Aging 20: 487–502
Vaupel J, Manton K, Stallard E (1979) The impact of heterogeneity in individual frailty on the dynamics of mortality. Demography 16: 439–454
West-Eberhard MJ (1987) Flexible strategy and social evolution. In: Itô Y, Brown JL, Kikkawa J (eds) Animal societies: theories and fact. Japan Sci. Soc. Press, Tokyo, pp 35–51
West-Eberhard MJ (1996) Wasp societies as microcosms for the study of development and evolution. In: Turillazzi S, West-Eberhard MJ (eds) Natural history and evolution of paper wasp. Oxford University Press, New York, pp 290–317
Winston ML (1987) The biology of the honey bee. Harvard University Press, Cambridge, Massachusetts

# A review of genes that act downstream of the DAF-16 FOXO transcription factor to influence the life span of *C. elegans*

*Coleen T. Murphy*[1]

## Summary

In the work we have described here (Murphy et al. 2003), an unbiased microarray analysis was used to identify transcriptional targets of the DAF-2/DAF-16 pathway, and the identified genes were tested for their individual contributions to longevity. Because we applied an unbiased method of gene expression profiling of a combination of multiple mutant alleles as well as a time course of RNAi treatment, resulting in data from over 70 arrays, we were able to significantly reduce the number of false positives. We found not only the very few previously identified DAF-16 targets but also many novel targets, and the previously described DBE and a new motif were overrepresented in the promoters of the genes. The diversity of the core set of downstream targets suggests that the coordination of expression through DAF-16 is critical in the regulation of longevity.

DAF-16, a FOXO-family transcription factor, influences the rate of aging of *C. elegans* in response to insulin/IGF-1 signaling. Using DNA microarray analysis, we found that DAF-16 affects the expression of a set of genes during early adulthood, the time at which this pathway is known to influence aging, and we have shown that many of these genes influence the aging process (Murphy et al. 2003). We also identified a DNA motif, in addition to the canonical DAF-16 motif, that is overrepresented in the promoters of the DAF-16-regulated genes. The insulin/IGF-1 pathway functions cell non-autonomously to regulate life span, and our findings suggest that it signals other cells, at least in part, by feedback regulation of two insulin/IGF-1 homologs.

Our findings suggest that the insulin/IGF-1 pathway ultimately exerts its effect on life span by up-regulating a wide variety of genes, including cellular stress response and anti-microbial genes, fat and steroid hormone synthesis genes, and many genes of unknown function, and by down-regulating specific life-shortening genes. Because the genes seem to act in a cumulative manner to affect life span, this study demonstrates the power of functional microarray analysis for dissecting complex regulatory systems.

*C. elegans* has proven to be an excellent model system for the study of aging. In addition to its general utility in genetic approaches (Brenner 1974), the worm also displays distinct phenotypes of aging during its short life span, allowing researchers to study long- and short-lived mutants (Johnson 1990; Kenyon et al. 1993; Lin

[1] University of California, San Francisco, CA

Carey et al.
Longevity and Frailty

et al. 1997; Lakowski and Hekimi 1996; Ewbank et al. 1997; Dillin et al. 2002a) as well as treatments that affect longevity (Lakowski and Hekimi 1998; Melov 2002). Two recent studies (Herndon et al. 2002; Garigan et al. 2002) carefully described the stochastic progression of aging in worms, which is marked by general tissue deterioration and reduction of motility. Age-related changes include sarcopenia, distortion of the cuticle, collapse and bacterial packing of the pharynx, distortion of gonadal nuclei, and the accumulation of fat in droplets in the head (Herndon et al. 2002; Garigan et al. 2002). Many of these phenotypes are reminiscent of human aging, and the fact that the genetic pathways known to affect life span in worms are highly conserved (Kenyon 2001; Guarente and Kenyon 2000) suggests that what we glean through studies of *C. elegans* aging will shed light on the mechanisms of aging regulation in humans.

Among the genetic mechanisms known to affect aging in *C. elegans*, the DAF-2/Insulin-IGF-like receptor (IIR) pathway (Kenyon et al. 1993) has perhaps the most dramatic effects and is one of the best studied. *daf-2* mutants are not only long-lived, with a life span of two to three times that of wild type worms, but the mutants are also extremely healthy and active much later than wild type (Kenyon et al. 1993). Many of the components of this signaling pathway have been cloned and characterized and include a PI3-kinase (*age-1*; Morris et al. 1996), a PTEN phosphatase (*daf-18*; Ogg and Ruvkun 1998), and additional kinases (*akt-1, akt-2, pdk-1*, and *sgk-1*; Paradis et al. 1999; Paradis and Ruvkun 1998; Hertwick et al. 2004). The activation of DAF-2/IIR activates this kinase cascade, culminating in the phosphorylation and nuclear exclusion of the DAF-16/FOXO transcription factor (Lin et al. 1997; Ogg et al. 1997; Lee et al. 2001). The activity of DAF-16/FOXO is required for all of the known phenotypes of *daf-2* mutants, including its extended longevity (Kenyon et al. 1993). However, the downstream targets of this transcription factor were largely unknown before the work we will describe here. Additionally, the only mechanism that had been hypothesized to function downstream of DAF-16/FOXO to extend life span involved the mediation of reactive oxygen species (Honda and Honda 1999). This paper will describe the work that we have done to discover these genes and test their roles in longevity. (For additional details and supplementary data, please see Murphy et al. 2003.)

## What are the transcriptional targets of DAF-16/FOXO?

### Previous work to identify the targets

Genetic screens to find genes downstream of DAF-16/FOXO were largely unsuccessful (Lin et al. 2001; Lee et al. 2002), identifying only genes that act in parallel to DAF-16, such as mitochondrial genes (Lee et al. 2002). One interpretation of these results is that, rather than acting through a single linear pathway, many genes may act in concert downstream of DAF-16.

A few DAF-16/FOXO target genes have been identified through candidate gene approaches. Because *daf-2* worms are not only long-lived but also exhibit resistance to oxidative stress, heat, and heavy metals, genes that might confer such resistance are good candidates for regulation by the DAF-2/DAF-16 pathway. Superoxide dismutase (*sod-3*; Honda and Honda 1999), a metallothionein (*mtl-1*; Barsyte et al. 2001), and a small heat-shock protein (*hsp-16;* Walker et al. 2001) were all shown to be upregulated in the long-lived *daf-2* or *age-1* mutants. The absence of these genes had not yet been shown to suppress *daf-2* life span, however, suggesting that additional targets remained.

## Our approach

Another method of identifying putative targets of a transcription factor is to find genes that contain the factor's binding site in the gene's promoter region. The DAF-16 binding element (DBE) TTGTTTAC had been identified by Furuyama et al. (2000) *in vitro*, so initially we looked for genes that contained the DBE within the first 1 kb upstream of the start site. We found that nearly one of every six promoters in the *C. elegans* genome contained a DBE. This number of genes seemed impractically high. [It should be noted, however, that in a simultaneous study, Lee et al. (2003) compared a list of DBE-containing *C. elegans* genes to a list of *Drosophila* orthologs that also contained this promoter element to obtain a smaller list of candidate DAF-16 targets to test.]

Because the principal role of DAF-16 is to control transcription, we decided to use expression analysis to identify the DAF-16/FOXO targets. We would like to point out some important points regarding our experimental approach that helped us to obtain a relatively small but significant group of DAF-2/DAF-16 targets:

1) unbiased selection of genes: we built full-genome *C. elegans* PCR microarrays for this analysis rather than examining a pre-defined set of genes;
2) predictive viewpoint: we looked at gene expression differences in early adulthood, before any aging or death has occurred, to identify differences that should **predict** the life span of the animal, rather than differences that are due to late aging;
3) biological redundancy and timecourse experiments: we used replicates of three alleles of *daf-2 (e1368, e1370*, and *mu150), age-1(hx546)*, and a DAF-16 overexpression strain compared with their respective *daf-16* double mutants or wild type background to identify DAF-2/DAF-16 differentially expressed genes that are shared between all of the long-lived strains. Ten of these experiments were included in the analysis.

   We also took advantage of the fact that in *C. elegans*, RNA interference is very simple; worms may be fed bacteria containing the double-stranded RNA of a gene of interest, and the gene's transcript will be knocked down. RNAi of *daf-2* recapitulates the long-lived phenotype of the *daf-2* mutant (Dillin et al. 2002b). We carried out two 10-point time courses of *daf-2* RNAi, *daf-2* + *daf-16* RNAi, and control vector treatment. Sixty arrays were included in this analysis. From these two experiments, we were able to obtain information about both the DAF-2/DAF-16 pathway and normal early aging. Time course analysis helps eliminate a problem that is common to many microarray experiments that rely on a single time point, that is, generation of false positives through the misinterpretation of slight differences in developmental timing. In general, by studying multiple alleles and RNAi treatments that share the trait we are interested in (i.e., long life span as a result of altered insulin signaling), as well as by biologically reversing the treatment (*daf-16* RNAi) and by using a time course, we were able to significantly reduce the number of false positives in our data set;

4) two independent analyses: we used two completely different methods to analyze our data. First, we submitted the 60 RNAi time course arrays and five of the mutant arrays to Cluster (Eisen et al. 1998) as a single data set; after hierarchical clustering, we were able to easily identify two groups of genes: Class 1 genes were upregulated under *daf-2(-)* conditions and downregulated under *daf-16(-)* conditions, whereas Class 2 genes met the opposite criteria. Because of the large number of arrays that we used for the experiment, genes that changed randomly were extremely obvious in the Cluster dendrogram, and these false positives did not cluster with our genes of interest. In fact, the Class 1 and 2 clusters contained fewer than 200 genes total. Additionally, we performed Significance Analysis of Microarrays (SAM) on the 10 mutant arrays and were able to find the set of genes that were consistently up- or downregulated. Most of the genes in the SAM list had already been identified through the Cluster analysis, but we did find some genes that had small but significant (consistent) expression changes in the mutants;
5) prioritization: by examining the data from the Cluster and SAM analyses, we were able to prioritize each gene according to a) its significance score from the mutant SAM analysis, b) its presence in the Class 1 or Class 2 cluster, c) its expression pattern under different conditions, and d) the consistency of the gene's expression within the cluster. The 250 genes were then placed into categories of 1 (best) through 6 (marginal);
6) testing the candidate target genes: we used RNAi to test each gene's contribution to the life span extension seen in *daf-2* mutants, starting with Priority Group 1 and working our way downwards. We tested 58 of the highest priority genes multiple times for their roles in longevity.

By taking these factors into account during the experimental set-up, rather than simply doing a small number of arrays of one *daf-2* allele at a single point, we were able to eliminate false positives and focus quickly on a small set of genes. Additionally, our system allows us to easily test the candidate genes for their functional significance.

## Our results

### Microarray analysis

Using Cluster to group genes with similar expression profiles, we were able to identify two major clusters of DAF-2/DAF-16-regulated genes (Fig. 1). The Class 1 genes are upregulated in the long-lived *daf-2* mutants and under *daf-2(RNAi)* conditions while dowregulated under *daf-16(RNAi)* conditions, and the Class 2 genes show the converse transcriptional profile. The previously identified targets

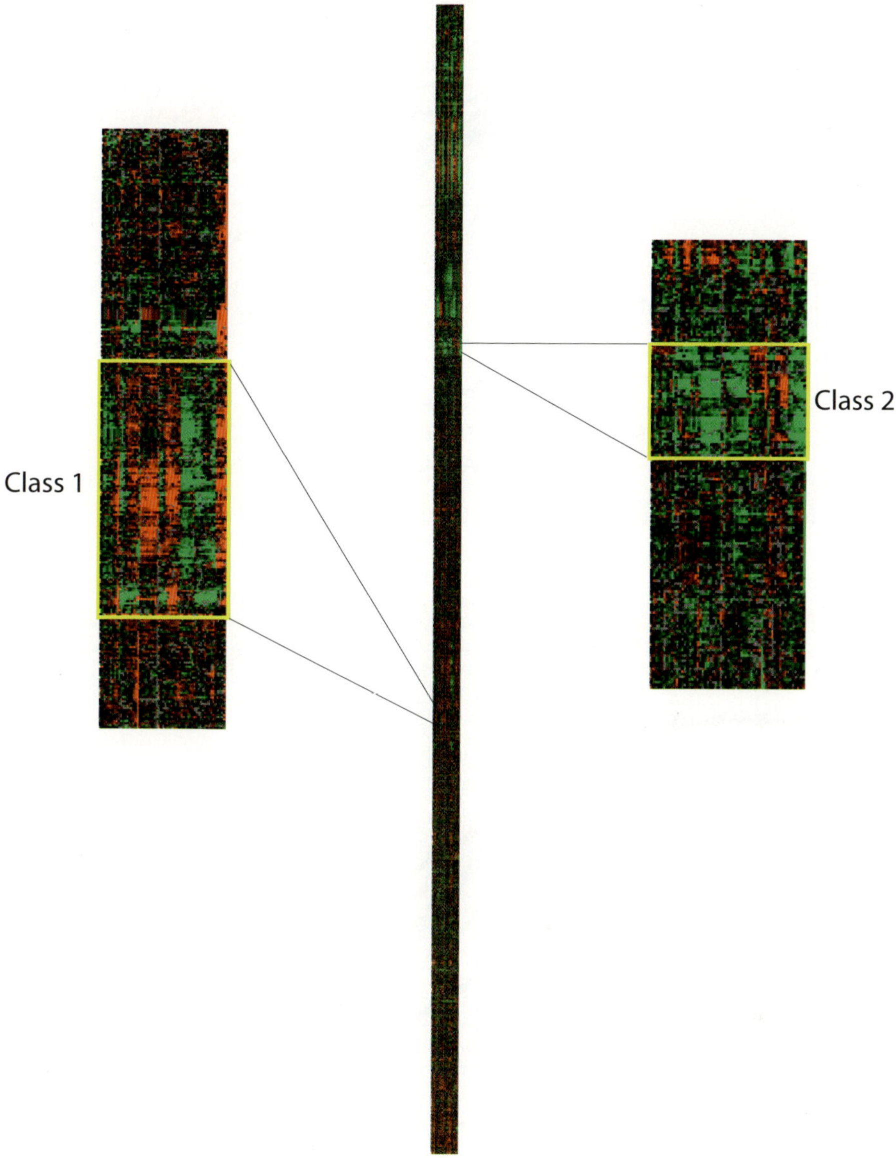


**Fig. 1.** Cluster of Class 1 and 2 genes. Many of the genes have a 10–20 % contribution to the lifespan of *daf-2* worms,while RNAi of *daf-16* is able to completely suppress longevity.

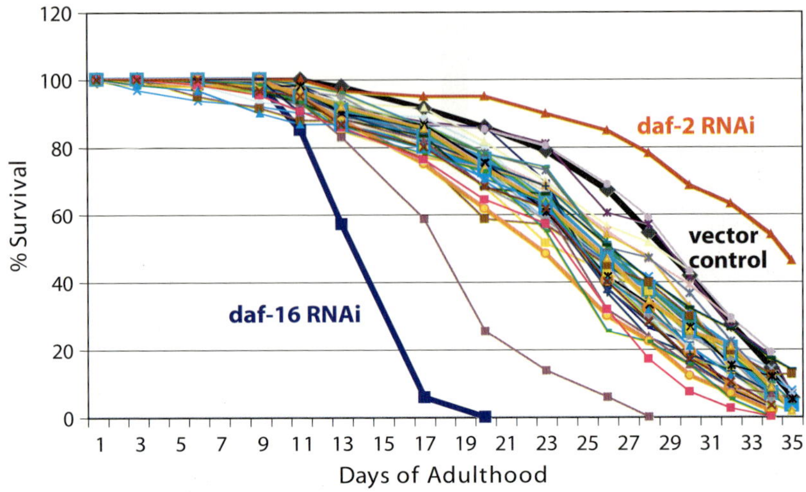


**Fig. 2.** Life span of *daf-2* worms on RNA interference of Class 1 genes.

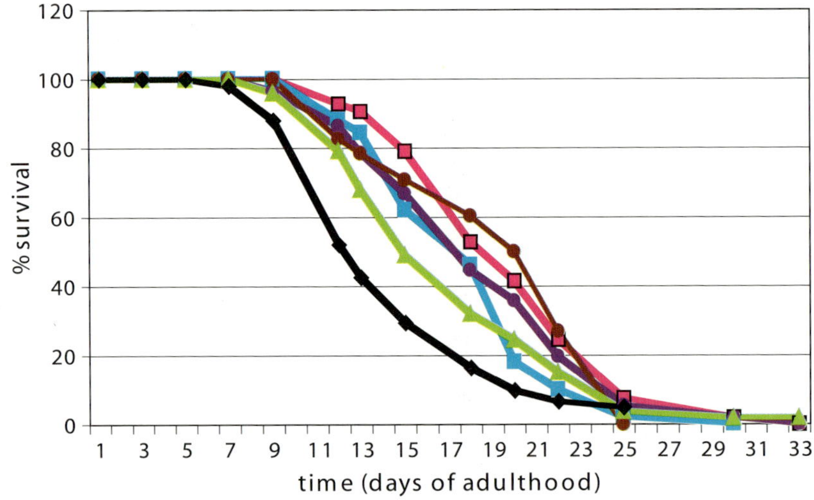


**Fig. 3.** Life span of wild type worms on RNA interference of Class 2 genes. RNAi of many of the Class 2 genes is able to increase the lifespan of wild type worms.

*sod-3, mtl-1,* and *hsp-16.2* were present in our Class 1 cluster, verifying our approach. Class 1 includes not only the expected genes involved in oxidative and heat stress response but also genes that function in activities not previously associated with prevention of aging in worms: antibacterials, cytochrome P450s, steroid and lipid synthesis, and specific metabolism genes. One of the 38 insulin-like peptide genes, *ins-18*, showed a small but significant increase in expression across all of the *daf-2* mutants. Additionally, novel genes, which we are naming *dod* for "downstream of DAF-16," were present in Class 1.

Class 2 includes genes involved in ubiquitin-mediated protein degradation *(skr)*, peptide transport, peptidases, apolipoproteins (vitellogenins), some neuronal (*gcy-6, gcy-18*) and signaling (*nhr*) molecules, and many novel genes. Additionally, *ins-7*, another insulin-like peptide gene, is significantly downregulated in *daf-2* worms. It should be noted that this is the first evidence that DAF-16 may play a direct role in gene repression.

Independent of the DAF-2/DAF-16-regulated genes, collagens and histones each show age-dependent changes, with collagen expression decreasing over time and histone expression increasing. Other early adult age-dependent expression is also apparent in our data.

## Promoter analysis

We examined the promoters of the Class 1 and Class 2 genes and found that the canonical DAF-16 binding element (DBE), with variation at the seventh nucleotide, was overrepresented, suggesting that many of the genes are indeed direct targets of DAF-16 transcription. Additionally, a novel element (the DAF-16-associated element, or DAE) with some similarity to the GATA transcriptional motif, was also overrepresented, suggesting the involvement of a co-factor or downstream transcription factor. Interestingly, both motifs are present in the promoters of both classes. Also, the presence of the DBE in the Class 2 genes suggests that DAF-16 is directly involved in these genes' repression.

## Life span analysis: RNAi of individual candidate genes

We were interested in establishing the contribution of each gene to *daf-2*'s long life span. To do this, we first prioritized the genes by the magnitude and consistency of expression changes. We then used feeding RNAi of the top genes first in life span tests, working our way down the priority list. Knockdown of many of the top-priority Class 1 genes shortened the life span of *daf-2* mutants (Fig. 2), whereas reduction of the lower priority genes had little to no effect. With the exception of T10B9.1, a cytochrome P450, reduction of most of the genes had no effect on wild type life span; RNAi of T10B9.1 affected development and dauer exit as well as shortening *daf-2*'s life span greatly. Another exception was B0213.15, also a cytochrome P450, which did not affect life span of wild type but extended *daf-2*'s life span significantly; this gene was the single exception to the general observation that RNAi of Class 1 genes either shortened or had no effect on *daf-2* life span. We also found that RNAi of many of the top-priority Class 2 genes extended the life span of wild type worms (Fig. 3), including the apolipoproteins, the *gcys*, several novel genes, and *ins-7*, which showed a very large increase in life span, reminiscent of *daf-2* RNAi treatment.

## Biological implications of our findings

Our results suggest that DAF-16 activity is important to the survival of *daf-2* mutants because it coordinates the expression of many different genes that may cumulatively contribute to longevity. The genes regulated by DAF-16 comprise a large number of functional classes, including stress response, antimicrobials, steroid synthesis, metabolism, lipid synthesis, apolipoproteins, protein and peptide degradation, and signaling. After identifying the genes downstream of DAF-16, we tested them individually for their life span effects, and we have shown here that many of the genes contribute individually to longevity. The wide variety of functions of life span-affecting genes emphasizes the importance of multiple systems in keeping the organism alive.

The presence of the DAF-16-binding element in the promoters of both Class 1 and Class 2 genes suggests that DAF-16 not only promotes but also represses expression of some genes. Additionally, the presence of the DAF-16-associated element (DAE) in these promoters suggests the activity of an additional co-factor or downstream signal.

The discovery of regulation of a pair of insulins, *ins-7* and *ins-18*, downstream of DAF-16 suggests the presence of a feed-forward mechanism that may coordinate the activity of the DAF-2 pathway in cells throughout the organism. This type of control could be especially important for longevity, since the survival of all the tissues is necessary for long life.

## Future directions

We looked for the targets of the DAF-2/DAF-16 pathway in early adulthood because we were interested in genes that are predictive of life span. Future experiments will tell us whether, at different times in the life of *C. elegans*, the activities of these genes have any bearing on longevity. While we have briefly mentioned some genes associated with general early aging, in the future it will be interesting to know all of the genes that change with late aging (Lund et al. 2002), as well as how DAF-16 target genes change with age.

It is not yet known whether there is an additional systemic pathway downstream of DAF-16. We can surmise that those genes with DBEs are direct targets of DAF-16, but our experiment does not distinguish direct from indirect targets. Later experiments will address this through biochemical techniques, including ChIP/chip analysis.

While the neurons were previously thought to be the primary site of DAF-2-mediated longevity control (Wolkow et al. 2000; Apfeld and Kenyon 1998, 1999), recent experiments with tissue-specific expression of DAF-16 suggest that the intestine may play a larger role in life span determination than previously appreciated (Libina et al. 2003). Our experiments were carried out on whole animals expressing DAF-16 in all tissues (or lacking DAF-16 in all tissues); it is possible that in the future we could dissect the pathway downstream of DAF-16 further by using strains expressing DAF-16 only in specific tissues.

Additionally, our microarray analyses were performed on populations of worms, to parallel our life span analyses, which are always done on populations as well. However, it would be interesting to combine the technique of single-worm microarray analysis[36] with the morphological analysis of aging (Herndon et al. 2002; Garigan et al. 2002). From this type of analysis we could obtain information about genes that change as an individual worm ages, and we could compare this information with that from our large-scale studies.

During our work, two other studies also looked for the downstream targets of DAF-16. As mentioned above, Lee et al. (2003) looked for genes that contained the in vitro-defined DBE and had orthologs with DBEs in flies. From this list they were able to find several targets that indeed were regulated in a DAF-2/DAF-16-dependent fashion and proved to have life span functions, as well. We have found an additional motif as well as a slight relaxation of the previously defined DBE in the promoters of our DAF-2/DAF-16 genes, and the genes with these motifs would not have been identified in the Lee et al. study. Thus, their approach, while avoiding many false positives and finding genuine targets that have life span effects, missed many other true DAF-16 targets.

A study by McElwee et al. (2003) also used microarrays to find targets of DAF-2/DAF-16. Their experiments were limited to four comparisons of one allele of *daf-2* with a *daf-16; daf-2* double mutant at a single time point, and they find thousands of genes varying between their samples. Due to this large number, they were unable to verify the life span contributions of the genes. In summary, we have used full-genome *C. elegans* microarrays to identify the downstream targets of the insulin/FOXO pathway, and we have tested these genes for their roles in longevity. This pathway is critical in the coordination of many genes that contribute to the lifespan of the organism.

## References

Apfeld J, Kenyon C (1998) Cell nonautonomy of *C. elegans daf-2* function in the regulation of diapause and life span. Cell 95: 199-210

Apfeld J, Kenyon C (1999) Regulation of life span by sensory perception in *Caenorhabditis elegans*. Nature 402: 804-809

Barsyte D, Lovejoy DA, Lithgow GJ (2001) Longevity and heavy metal resistance in *daf-2* and *age-1* long-lived mutants of *Caenorhabditis elegans*. FASEB J 15: 627-634

Brenner S (1974) The genetics of *Caenorhabditis elegans*. Genetics 77: 71-94

Dillin A, Hsu AL, Arantes-Oliveira N, Lehrer-Graiwer J, Hsin H, Fraser AG, Kamath RS, Ahringer J, Kenyon C (2002) Rates of behavior and aging specified by mitochondrial function during development. Science 298: 2398-2401

Dillin A, Crawford DK, Kenyon C (2002) Timing requirements for insulin/IGF-1 signaling in *C. elegans*. Science 298: 830-834

Eisen MB, Spellman PT, Brown PO, Botstein D (1998) Cluster analysis and display of genome-wide expression patterns. Proc Natl Acad Sci USA 95:14863-14868

Ewbank JJ, Barnes TM, Lakowski B, Lussier M, Bussey H, Hekimi S (1997) Structural and functional conservation of the Caenorhabditis elegans timing gene *clk-1*. Science 275: 980-983

Furuyama T, Nakazawa T, Nakano I, Mori N (2000) Identification of the differential distribution patterns of mRNAs and consensus binding sequences for mouse DAF-16 homologues. Biochem J 349: 629-634

Garigan D, Hsu AL, Fraser AG, Kamath RS, Ahringer J, Kenyon C (2002) Genetic analysis of tissue aging in *Caenorhabditis elegans*. A role for heat-shock factor and bacterial proliferation. Genetics 161: 1101-1112

Golden T.R, Melov S (2004) Microarray analysis of gene expression with age in individual nematodes. Aging Cell 3: 111-124

Guarente L, Kenyon C (2000) Genetic pathways that regulate ageing in model organisms. Nature 408: 255-262

Herndon LA, Schmeissner PJ, Dudaronek JM, Brown PA, Listner KM, Sakano Y, Paupard MC, Hall DH, Driscoll M (2002) Stochastic and genetic factors influence tissue-specific decline in ageing *C. elegans*. Nature 419: 808-814

Hertwick M, Goebel C, Baumeister R (2004) C. elegans SGK-1 is the critical component in the Akt/PKB kinase complex to control stress response and life span. Dev Cell 8: 577-588

Honda Y, Honda S (1999) The *daf-2* gene network for longevity regulates oxidative stress resistance and Mn-superoxide dismutase gene expression in *Caenorhabditis elegans*. FASEB J 13: 1385-1393

Johnson TE (1990) Increased life-span of age-1 mutants in Caenorhabditis elegans and lower Gompertz rate of aging. Science 249: 908-912

Kenyon C (2000) A conserved regulatory system for aging. Cell 105: 165-168

Kenyon C, Chang J, Gensch E, Rudner A, Tabtiang R (1993) A *C. elegans* mutant that lives twice as long as wild type. Nature 366: 461-464

Lakowski,B, Hekimi S (1996) Determination of life-span in Caenorhabditis elegans by four clock genes. Science 272: 1010-1013

Lakowski B, Hekimi S (1998) The genetics of caloric restriction in *Caenorhabditis elegans*. Proc Natl Acad Sci USA 95: 13091-13096

Lee RY, Hench J, Ruvkun G (2001) Regulation of *C. elegans* DAF-16 and its human ortholog FKHRL1 by the *daf-2* insulin-like signaling pathway. Curr Biol 11: 1950-1957

Lee SS, Lee RYN, Fraser AG, Kamath RS, Ahringer J, Ruvkun G (2002) A systematic RNAi screen identifies a critical role for mitochondria in *C. elegans* longevity. Nature Genet 33: 40-48

Lee SS, Kennedy S, Tolonen AC, Ruvkun G (2003) DAF-16 target genes that control C. elegans life-span and metabolism. Science 300: 644-647

Libina N, Berman JR, Kenyon C (2003) Tissue-specific activities of *C. elegans* DAF-16 in the regulation of life span. Cell 115: 489-502

Lin K, Dorman JB, Rodan A, Kenyon C (1997) *daf-16*: An HNF-3/forkhead family member that can function to double the life-span of *Caenorhabditis elegans*. Science 278: 1319-1322

Lin K, Hsin H, Libina N, Kenyon C (2001) Regulation of the *Caenorhabditis elegans* longevity protein DAF-16 by insulin/IGF-1 and germline signaling. Nature Genet 28: 139-145

Lund J, Tedesco P, Duke K, Wang J, Kim SK, Johnson TE (2002) Transcriptional profile of aging in *C. elegans*. Curr Biol 12: 1566-1573

McElwee J, Bubb K, Thomas JH (2003) Transcriptional outputs of the *Caenorhabditis elegans* forkhead transcription protein DAF-16. Aging Cell 2: 111-121

Melov S (2002) Therapeutics against mitochondrial oxidative stress in animal models of aging. Ann NY Acad Sci 959: 330-340

Morris JZ, Tissenbaum HA, Ruvkun G (1996) A phosphatidylinositol-3-OH kinase family member regulating longevity and diapause in *Caenorhabditis elegans*. Nature 382: 536-539

Murphy CT, McCarroll A, Bargmann I, Fraser A, Kamath R, Ahringer J, Kenyon C (2003) Genes that act downstream of DAF-16 to influence the life span of *Caenorhabditis elegans*. Nature 424: 277-283

Ogg S, Ruvkun G (1998) The C. elegans PTEN homolog, DAF-18, acts in the insulin receptor-like metabolic signaling pathway. Mol Cell 2: 887-893

Ogg S, Paradis S, Gottlieb S, Patterson GI, Lee L, Tissenbaum HA, Ruvkun G (1997) The Fork head transcription factor DAF-16 transduces insulin-like metabolic and longevity signals in *C. elegans*. Nature 389: 994-999

Paradis S, Ruvkun G (1998) *Caenorhabditis elegans* Akt/PKB transduces insulin receptor-like signals from AGE-1 PI3 kinase to the DAF-16 transcription factor. Genes Dev 12: 2488-2498

Paradis S, Ailion M, Toker A, Thomas JH, Ruvkun G (1999) A PDK1 homolog is necessary and sufficient to transduce AGE-1 PI3 kinase signals that regulate diapause in *Caenorhabditis elegans*. Genes Dev 13: 1438-1452

Walker GA, White TM, McColl G, Jenkins NL, Babich S, Candido EP, Johnson TE, Lithgow GJ (2001) Heat shock protein accumulation is upregulated in a long-lived mutant of Caenorhabditis elegans. J Gerontol A Biol Sci Med Sci 56: B281-287

Wolkow CA, Kimura KD, Lee MS, Ruvkun G (2000) Regulation of *C. elegans* life-span by insulin-like signaling in the nervous system. Science 290: 147-150

# Calorie restriction in nonhuman primates: impact on aging, disease, and frailty

*Donald K. Ingram[1], Rafael de Cabo, R. Michael Anson, Mary Ann Ottinger[2], Mark A. Lane[3], George S. Roth, Julie A. Mattison*

## Summary

Dietary caloric restriction (CR) is the only intervention repeatedly demonstrated to retard the onset and incidence of age-related diseases, maintain function, and extend both life span and health span in mammals. In 70 years of study, such beneficial effects have been demonstrated in rodents and lower animals but, prior to 1987, had never been examined in primates. To determine whether CR might eventually be applied to humans, the NIA initiated a study of CR and aging in nonhuman primates. After nearly 18 years, male and female rhesus monkeys (*Macaca mulatta*) of different ages have been involved in the study, including many old monkeys begun on CR (>15 yrs). Systematic CR studies of older individuals from long-lived species have not been conducted to date. Control monkeys receive two meals per day, sufficient to attain apparent satiety, whereas the CR group receives 30% less, adjusted for age and body weight. The diet is supplemented with extra micronutrients such that the only substantive variable is the amount of calories consumed. Based on results observed to date, rhesus monkeys exhibit many CR-associated beneficial effects that resemble those observed in CR rodents, such as decreased fat, improved glucoregulatory function, and decreased risk factors for cardiovascular disease and diabetes. Results produced thus far demonstrate that older monkeys can respond to a 30% CR in a manner similar to young animals. For some variables, such as loss of fat, older monkeys do not respond as well. For other variables, such as increased production of melatonin, older monkeys respond more robustly than do young monkeys. Current analyses do not indicate any beneficial or detrimental effects of this nutritional regimen on rates of mortality and morbidity among older monkeys. For selected variables, such as bone density, further analyses will be needed to assess whether CR will have detrimental effects on aging. Additional assessment of the patterns of individual aging among the older cohorts of monkeys will also permit characterization of frailty and factors that predispose monkeys to frailty.

---

[1] Correspondence should be sent to Donald K. Ingram, Acting Chief, Laboratory of Experimental Gerontology, Gerontology Research Center, National Institute on Aging, NIH, 5600 Nathan Shock Drive, Baltimore, MD 21224, Phone: 410-558-8180; Fax: 410-558-8302; E-mail: ingramd@grc.nia.nih.gov.

[2] Department of Avian and Animal Science, University of Maryland, College Park, MD 20742

[3] Current address: Merck and Company, Rahway, NJ 07065

Carey et al.
Longevity and Frailty

## Introduction

Over the last few decades, numerous studies in laboratory rodents (Masoro 2000; Weindruch and Walford 1988; Yu 1994) have demonstrated that the most robust means of decelerating the rate of aging is calorie restriction (CR). When consumption of a nutritious diet is reduced 30–50% from control levels beginning in juvenile or even young adult animals, CR study results include observations of increased life span, decreased incidence and delayed onset of age-related diseases, increased resistance to various stressors, and extended maintenance of physiological and behavioral function (Masoro 2000; Weindruch and Walford 1988; Yu 1994).

Despite the abundant evidence indicating the benefits of CR on aging processes in young animals, little systematic research has been conducted to assess the benefits or risks of CR initiated in old animals. A recent report in mice (Dhahbi et al. 2004) indicated that initiation of 40% CR in middle-aged mice (male B6C3F$_1$, 18 months of age) resulted in significantly increased life span as well as a pattern of gene expression resembling that observed in younger mice. However, such reports of CR effects in older animals have not always been so consistent. For example, Forster et al. (2003) reported that 40% CR initiated in old mice (22–24 months) increased mortality in three mouse strains, especially in DBA/2J mice. In fact, switching from CR to an ad libitum (AL) diet was beneficial for survival of these aged mice. Similarly, Goodrick et al. (1990) reported that CR induced by every-other-day (EOD) feeding in male mice from three strains produced no significant effects on life span in two strains when initiated at 18 months of age and actually reduced life span in A/J mice.

The relevance of CR to human aging is still emerging. Few systematic studies have been conducted in humans that did not involve near starvation or extremely low calorie diets. The Biosphere experiment represents one of the most comprehensive studies approximating CR in man (Verdery et al. 1998; Walford et al. 1992, 2002). Biosphere 2 was a closed environment in the Arizona desert that housed, over a two-year period, four male and four female occupants aged 27–42, with one 67-year-old. The average food intake for much of the two years was estimated to be 1,800 kcal/day and was essentially the same for all occupants, regardless of sex or body weight. Their overall intake approximated a 30% CR. Results indicated that physiological responses to CR in this group of humans appeared similar to those reported in rodents: specifically, body weight, fasting glucose, serum cholesterol and triglycerides, and blood pressure were all reduced.

A recent report has examined a group of adults (35–82 years; mean age = 50 years) who were on self-imposed CR for extended periods of time (mean duration = six years) compared to a group of control subjects of similar age who were not dieting (Fontana et al. 2004). Results clearly indicated a reduction in risk factors for cardiovascular disease among the CR practitioners, including reduced cholesterol, glucose, insulin, blood pressure, C-reactive protein and intima-media thickness of the carotid artery. Many years ago, an interesting study was conducted among nursing home residents in Spain. Vallejo (1957) noted that, when residents (>65 years) were provided a regimen of EOD feeding that reduced caloric intake compared to a control group fed daily, the number of sick days in the CR group and the number of deaths over a three-year period were reduced (Vallejo 1957).

To provide a more systematic experimental approach, the National Institute on Aging (NIA) is sponsoring three clinical trials of CR at the Pennington Nutrition Research Center, Louisiana State University, Washington University, and the Tufts University Jean Mayer Human Nutrition Research Center on Aging (Heilbroon and Ravussin 2003). Each of these centers is taking a slightly different approach to their studies in regard to the CR regimens and the endpoints, and one of them is examining the intervention in older persons (Washington University).

The relevance of CR to long-lived species, particularly to humans, is being addressed in studies of rhesus monkeys at the Wisconsin National Primate Research Center (WNPRC) and at the National Institute on Aging (NIA). The advantages of using rhesus monkeys for studies of aging and human health interventions have been reported recently (Roth et al. 2004). Both the WNPRC and the NIA studies are accumulating data on mortality and morbidity as well as examining a wide range of parameters from cellular to functional levels to determine if 30% CR can retard the rate of aging (Ingram et al. 1990; Kemnitz et al. 1993; Wanagat et al. 1999). The WNPRC study was initiated in 1989 and now involves both male and female monkeys first introduced to 30% CR as adults (8–14 years of age). The NIA study was initiated in 1987 and involves male and female monkeys maintained on a highly nutritious control (CON) diet or introduced to CR of the same diet at different stages of their life span, including juvenile (one to three years), adult (4–13 years), and old (15–23 years). Median life span in rhesus monkeys is estimated to be 25 years, with a maximum of 40 years (Colman and Kemnitz 1998; Jones 1968; Wood 1991). Also included in the NIA study are smaller cohorts of monkeys (n=5–8) that were begun on CR as young (four to six years) or old (15–24 years) adults, many of which are now housed at the Oregon National Primate Research Center (ONPRC), where a variety of assays are being conducted with primary emphasis on 24-hr sampling of hormones.

Details of the husbandry and diet used in the NIA study have been presented in detail elsewhere (Ingram et al. 1990). In general, the regimen involves a nutritionally fortified semi-purified diet that is low in fat (5%) and protein (15%) and high in fiber (7%). CR monkeys are provided a food allotment that represents 30% fewer calories than that given to age- and weight-matched CON monkeys. This level of restriction was instituted gradually, with a 10% drop per month for three months. Similarly, CR was instituted over a three-month period in monkeys housed at ONPRC; however, food allotments were calculated as 30% less than an individual monkey's control consumption. Monkeys at both locations were offered two meals daily: one in the morning and one in the early afternoon.

Although the NIA study is still in progress, 17 years of data allow us to address the impact of CR on many aspects of aging, disease, and frailty. In addition, we can focus on CR imposed on older animals to determine if this is a healthy intervention applicable to human aging.

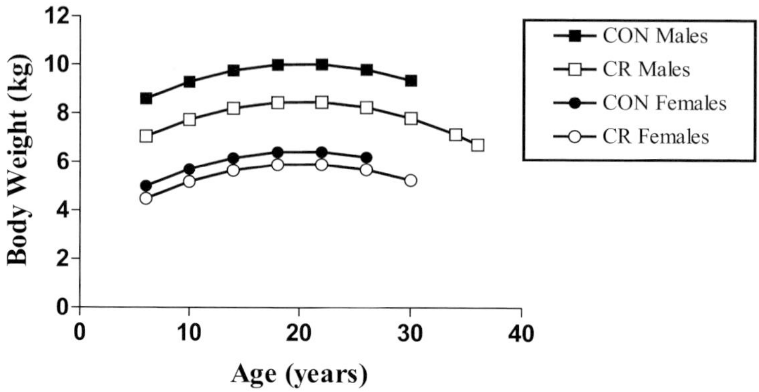


**Fig. 1.** Mixed effects model of body weight of rhesus monkeys on a control (CON) diet or on the same diet as 30% calorie restriction (CR).

## Body Mass and Composition

It is not surprising that a 30% CR regimen can reduce body weight and fat composition in young monkeys, but what about in older ones? Figure 1 shows a mixed effect model of body mass as a function of age greater than six years for all monkey groups (Mattison et al. 2004). Data available from the earliest ages indicate that rhesus monkeys continue to gain weight throughout adulthood, but a decline is evident by the age of 25. Also apparent is that male monkeys respond to CR to a notably greater extent than do females. Figure 2 presents estimates of percentage of fat as measured by dual beam X-ray absorbitometry (DEXA) for groups of monkeys begun on CR as juveniles or young adults versus those started as old adults. Again female responses to CR in terms of fat loss were less than those observed in males, and the older monkeys lost less fat than did younger cohorts. Indeed, there was no detectable loss in females after the first measurement.

A shorter-term study involving 12 male rhesus monkeys (18–25 years of age) showed that reduced body weight and fat were clearly obtainable with a 30% CR imposed gradually, with a 10% reduction each month. Figure 3 presents these results, indicating that reductions of over 20% in body weight and 40% in fat could be reached after a year on the diet in this old group of monkeys.

## Food Intake

An issue affecting the imposition of CR in older monkeys is the notable age-related loss of body weight accompanied by a steady decline in food intake. Figure 4 presents longitudinal estimates of daily caloric consumption of all monkeys based on a mixed effects model (Mattison et al., in press). In both males and females, there is clear decline in caloric intake that begins after maturity. There is notable convergence of intake between CON and CR monkeys for both males and females.

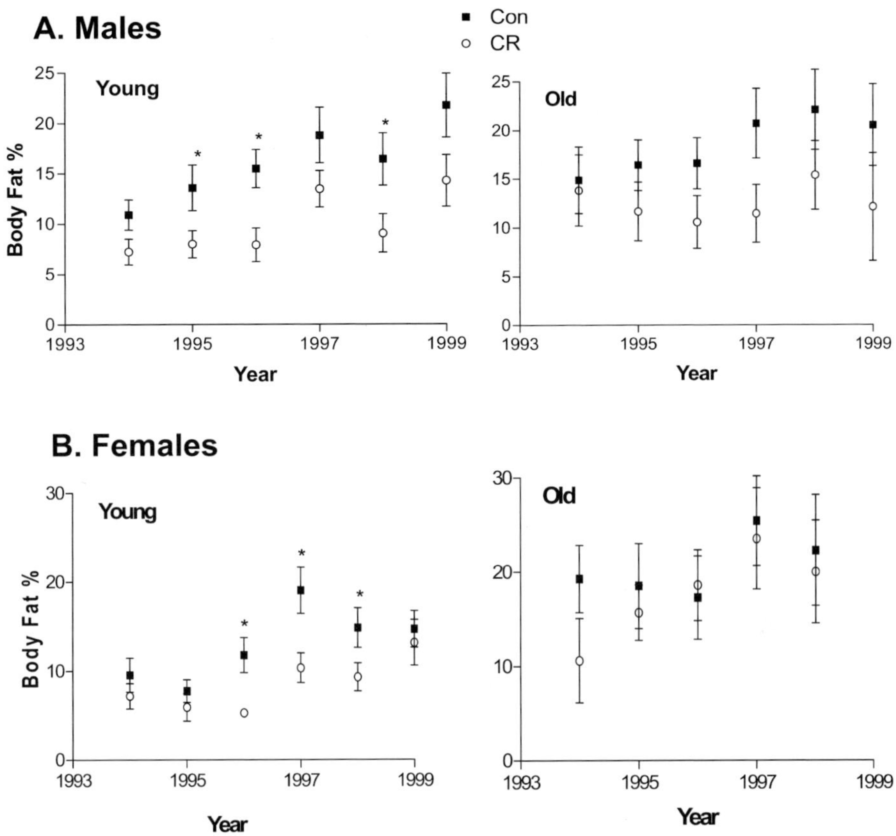


**Fig. 2.** Percent body fat in male (**A**) and female (**B**) rhesus monkeys on a control (CON) diet or on the same diet as 30% calorie restriction (CR).

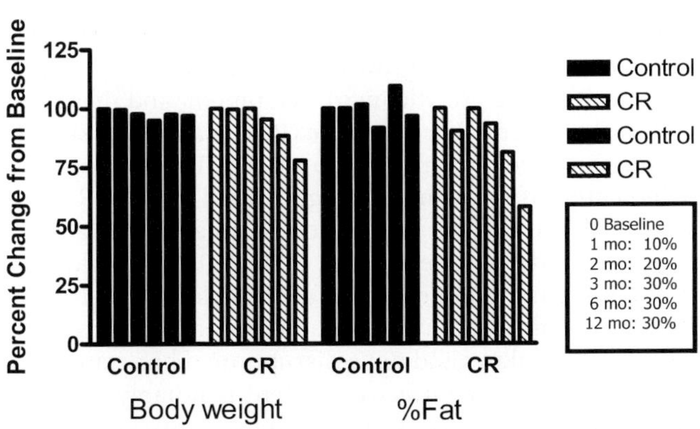


**Fig. 3.** Body weight and percent body fat change in male rhesus monkeys maintained on control diet or gradually introduced to CR at 18-25 years of age.

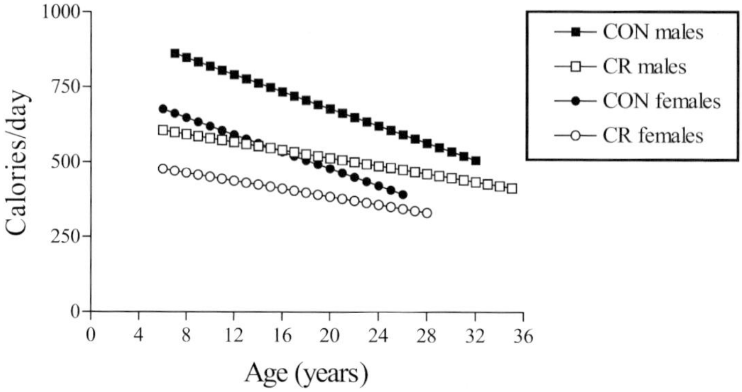


**Fig. 4.** Estimated daily caloric intake of adult rhesus monkeys on control (CON) or calorie restricted (CR) diets as a function of age.

In an evaluation of motivation for food, an age-related decline in the persistence with which monkeys attempted to retrieve a food reward was observed in CON monkeys in the NIA study (Mattison et al. 2004). Thus, at ages beyond 20 years, it is evident that imposition of 30% CR would be based on quite different baseline consumption and levels of appetite, which could prove to be less than optimal for the health of some animals. Because of this age-related decline in appetite, the feeding procedure for CR monkeys in the NIA has been to maintain the level of food offered to them at the highest level that they were provided during the study.

## Skeletal Aging

Reports from the NIA study have documented reduced or delayed skeletal development in young monkeys, as evidenced by shorter crown-rump measures in CR males compared to CON and an attenuation of the decline in serum alkaline phosphatase (AP), an osteoblastic product, in fully grown monkeys (Lane et al. 1995). Total AP levels are correlated with bone growth and development, and these levels bottom out at the age when bone growth is complete (Pyle et al. 1971), similar to the pattern observed in human development (Gordon 1993). This CR-induced delay in monkeys may be indicative of a slowing of an age-related process. Rodent studies also reported that CR delayed skeletal maturation (Kalu et al. 1984a,b).

Based on DEXA scanning of the NIA monkeys, Black et al. (2001) reported lower bone mineral content and bone mineral density in adult males after 11 years on CR compared to CON. These differences in male monkeys can be accounted for by lower body mass of the CR monkeys and not a disruption of bone turnover (Black et al. 2001). Similarly, femoral bone mineral content is notably lower in CR rats, which was also related to the reduction in body weight (Sanderson et al. 1997). Nonetheless, a CR effect on bone integrity is not without potential risk, as smaller body size and lower bone mineral density are associated with increased risk of fragility fractures in humans (De Laet et al. 1998; Ensrud et al. 1997). No detrimental effects have been evident in the NIA study to date.

In contrast to changes observed in male monkeys in the NIA study, bone mass in adult CR female monkeys has been maintained with advancing age, compared to CON female monkeys (Lane et al. 2001). This discrepancy in findings across gender may be explained by the older mean and maximum ages of the male population or by the fact that males were studied after 11 years on CR compared to only six years for the females; thus, additional research will be required with a particular focus on females as they enter menopausal ages. However, yearly measurements of biochemical markers of bone turnover or hormonal regulators of bone metabolism, such as osteoclacin, 25-hydroxyvitamin D, 1,25-hydroxyvitamin D, and parathyroid hormone, are not consistent with a greater active bone loss in the female CR monkeys (Lane et al. 2001). Similarly, bone mineral content and density are lower in CR monkeys at WNPRC compared to their controls, presumably due to their lower body weight. Measures of bone turnover have not been influenced by diet (Ramsey et al. 2000).

## Reproductive Function

When CR is imposed early in the life of male rhesus monkeys, puberty is delayed by about a year, based on measures of circulating testosterone (Roth et al. 1993). A similar finding has been observed in CR rodents (Merry and Holehan 1981) and undernourished humans (Bongaarts 1980). It is unknown whether this delay in sexual maturation, as observed for delayed skeletal maturation in CR animals, will predict increased life span.

If total and free testosterone decline with age in human males, such observations could be linked to other age-associated changes, such as decreased fat mass and muscle strength, bone loss, and the development of central obesity (Tenover 1997). A significant age-related decline in circulating testosterone has not been detected in the NIA study from either cross-sectional or longitudinal measures. Schwartz and Kemnitz (1992) reported a trend toward lower testosterone levels in male rhesus monkeys over 20 years of age, but due to the low sample size, the difference was also not significant. Kaler et al. (1986) noted similar levels in mean 24-hour plasma testosterone between young and old monkeys, but the pulsatile pattern of secretion differed between age groups. Testosterone concentration varies widely among individuals and throughout the day, so it is difficult to eliminate the marked variability, even with controlled sampling time. Currently, studies with monkeys at the ONPRC are being conducted using 24-hr blood sampling that will permit a clearer understanding of how CR and aging affect changes in testosterone concentration in these animals.

In female rhesus monkeys, the pattern of reproductive senescence is similar to the human experience (Lane et al. 2001; Black and Lane 2002). Hormonal changes leading to menopause are accompanied by changes in mood, skin and body composition, loss of bone mass, cognitive impairment, and increased risk for cardiovascular disease in both humans and rhesus monkeys (Lindsay et al. 1996). Thus, the rhesus monkey can be considered a valuable model for the study of menopause. Furthermore, CR intervention has been reported to attenuate the age-related decline in reproductive function in aging rats (Holehan and Merry 1985).

In analyses conducted to date, the NIA study has documented age-related hormonal differences in female monkeys aged 7–27 years that parallel some of the changes observed in previous studies in monkeys as well as in humans. Specifically, Lane et al. (2001) noted a significant, age-related decrease in both number and length of menstrual cycles, accompanied by a decline in serum estradiol and an increase in follicle stimulating hormone (FSH). Levels of progesterone decreased with age whereas leuteinizing hormone (LH) increased, but neither of these trends was statistically significant. In contrast to findings in rodent studies, none of these hormonal parameters were significantly altered by six years of 30% CR. The more moderate CR imposed in monkeys, 30% compared to 40% in rodents, might explain this species discrepancy in response. Moreover, rodents have an estrus cycle of only four to five days compared to the 24- to 31-day menstrual cycle observed in rhesus monkeys and humans. In addition, Black et al. (unpublished data) have shown that short-term (four-months) 30% CR did not alter ovulation in eight-year-old rhesus monkeys, indicating that the diet provided in the NIA study appears adequate to support ovulatory function. Current studies being conducted at NIA and ONPRC are examining this question, using more frequent blood sampling as well as *in vitro* fertilization techniques to directly evaluate fertility as affected by long-term CR.

## Glucoregulation

Similar to findings in rodent studies, CR has been shown to improve glucoregulation in primates. Rodent (Koizumi et al. 1989; Masoro et al. 1983; Reaven et al. 1983) and monkey studies (Kemnitz et al. 1994; Lane et al. 1995) document the effectiveness of CR in lowering fasting glucose and insulin levels. The glucose response of young monkeys in the NIA study appeared to be delayed by several years; reduced levels of fasting glucose were not reported at first (Cutler et al. 1992) but were noted later after three years of CR (Lane et al. 1995). This delay in glucose reduction appeared consistent with findings in the WNPRC study (Kemnitz et al. 1994), but such delays have not been reported as frequently in rodent studies. This species difference may be due to differences in body composition, relative percentage of life span on CR, diet composition, the severity of CR, or the techniques used to collect the blood samples (Lane et al. 1995). Figure 5A presents the fasting glucose data from the group of old male monkeys subjected to CR initiated at 18–25 years of age. There is a significant linear decline of about 20% in fasting glucose levels that took several months to appear but is apparent at one year into the study.

Plasma insulin levels, both at baseline and in response to an intravenous glucose challenge, are also reduced in adult CR monkeys (Lane et al. 1995). Moreover, the change in insulin levels is more robust than that of glucose even in older monkeys. Figure 5B shows the change in fasting insulin in old male monkeys gradually subjected to CR, with a nearly 50% reduction in plasma insulin evident after one year of 30% CR (Lane et al. 2000). Following a glucose challenge, aged

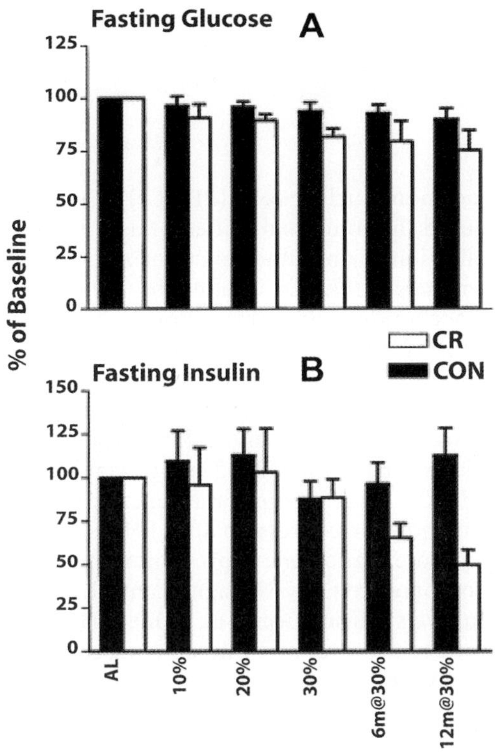


**Fig. 5.** Percent change from baseline in plasma glucose and insulin levels in male rhesus monkeys maintained on control (CON) diet or gradually introduced to CR at 18-25 years of age.

monkeys respond in a manner indicative of increased insulin receptor sensitivity (Lane et al. 2000). Such results indicate that CR could reduce the risk or postpone the onset of type II diabetes.

## Cardiovascular Function

Parameters of cardiovascular function and concomitant risk of cardiovascular disease have been assessed in monkeys in the NIA and WNPRC studies. Age-related differences in blood pressure have not been evident in the NIA study; however, Lane et al. (1998) reported significantly lower blood pressure in females after three years on CR compared to CON.

Measures of blood lipids in CR monkeys have suggested reduced risks for cardiovascular disease. In the NIA study, significant decreases in plasma triglycerides and an increase in the level of larger high-density lipoprotein fractions have been noted (Verdery et al. 1997). In the WNPRC study, reduced levels of lipoprotein (a) as well reduced interaction of low-density lipoproteins with proteoglycans have been reported (Edwards et al. 1998). In the NIA study of CR induced in 18- to 25-year-old male monkeys, triglycerides were reduced around 50% after one year of study, but total cholesterol and blood pressure were not markedly changed (Lane et al. 2000).

## Immune Function

Cytokine responses of peripheral blood mononuclear cells (PBMCs) to various inflammatory stimuli have been measured in monkeys of different ages in both the NIA and WNPRC studies as a reflection of immune function. Age-related increases in the production of inflammatory cytokines, interleukin (IL)-10 and IL-6 proteins in response to lipopolysaccharide (LPS) stimulation and an age-related decline in phytohaemagglutinin (PHA)-stimulated production of interferon-gamma (IFNγ) have been reported in the NIA study (Mascarucci et al. 2001). These findings indicated an age-related dysregulation of cytokine levels. To investigate the effects of CR on age-related changes in cytokine production, PBMCs from CON and CR rhesus monkeys aged 6–7 and 22–25 years were examined. Assays were conducted to assess IL-10 and IL-6 protein and gene expression after exposure to LPS, and IFNγ protein and gene expression after PHA stimulation. Significantly higher levels of IFNγ protein and gene expression were found in aged monkeys on CR for two years compared to CON. No significant CR effects were observed in IL-10 and IL-6 protein levels (Mascarucci et al. 2002). IFNγ plays a role in the initial defense mechanism against viral and microbial disease and cancer; thus, CR monkeys may benefit from this alteration in immune function.

Immunological results from the WNPRC study have been restricted to younger adult monkeys. However, findings published thus far indicate that concanavalin A and pokeweed mitogen response were reduced in CR monkeys; there was also a reduction in natural killer cell activity and the antibody response to influenza (Roecker et al. 1996). In a subsequent study, WNPRC reported a reduction in peripheral blood lymphocyte number over seven years of sampling in both CON and CR monkeys (Weindruch et al. 1997). Additional studies of immune function are ongoing at both NIA and WNPRC to clarify the effects of age and diet.

## Brain and Behavior

Two separate analyses of locomotor activity in the home cage have been conducted in the NIA study, but only one contained data on the effects of CR in old monkeys. Weed et al. (1997) reported an age-related decline in locomotor activity in adult male monkeys, with increased activity observed in CR monkeys compared to controls at 10–12 years of age. Examining a broader age range of female monkeys (6–26 years), Moscrip et al. (2000) recorded significant age-related decline in locomotor activity. CR monkeys in the youngest age group (6–10 years) showed significantly reduced daytime activity, but there were no significant effects on activity of CR in an old group of monkeys (18–27 years).

An age-related decline in the volume of the neostriatum is a well-established biomarker of brain aging in both humans (Krishnan et al. 1990; Murphy et al. 1992; Raz et al. 1995) and rhesus monkeys (Matochik et al. 2000) that may reflect diminished motor abilities in older individuals. A recent analysis of this structural change using magnetic imaging resonance (MRI) was conducted on male monkeys from the NIA study (Matochik et al. 2004). While significant age-related decreases in the relative volume of both the putamen and caudate nucleus were noted, there was no significant CR-related attenuation of this decline observed, even among older male monkeys. This analysis will be repeated over the next few years. In addition to measuring this change in brain structure, the monkeys are also being examined by positron emission tomography (PET) imaging to assess the age-related decline in the concentration of dopamine $D_2$ receptors in the same brain region. In a study utilizing only the control male monkeys in the NIA study, Morris et al. (1999) reported a significant decline in binding of these receptors in the striatum.

## Biomarkers of Aging

One on the objectives of the NIA study was to develop a strategy for identifying and validating biomarkers of aging. Details of this strategy have been published previously and include construction of a biological age score that could be used to assess whether an intervention can slow the rate of aging (Nakamura et al. 1994, 1998; Ingram et al. 2001). The basic features of this strategy were to identify variables that met the following statistical criteria: 1) significant cross-sectional correlation with age; 2) significant longitudinal change with age consistent with the cross-sectional correlation; 3) significant stability of individual differences over time; and 4) rate of age-related change in the biomarker is proportional to differences in life span among related species.

Dehydroepiandrosterone-sulfate (DHEAS), an adrenal steroid, has emerged as a strong candidate for a biomarker of aging. Major age-related declines in the serum level of this hormone have been reported in cross-sectional (Orentreich et al. 1984; Ohasi et al. 1986; Leblhuber et al. 1991) and longitudinal (Thomas et al. 1994; Orentreich et al. 1992) human studies. Elevated serum levels of DHEAS have been related to increased protection against age-associated diseases, such as diabetes (Small et al. 1989), heart disease (Barrett-Connor et al. 1986), and cancer (Zumoff et al. 1981).

A marked age-related decline in serum DHEAS has also been documented in rhesus monkeys. Kemnitz et al. (2000) reported about a 90% reduction in DHEAS from infancy through three years of age, followed by a more gradual decline, averaging 4.2% per year. DHEAS also showed this marked decline in adult rhesus monkeys in the NIA study according to a study by Lane et al. (1997). This study also demonstrated longitudinal change in DHEAS in rhesus monkeys and the significant stability of the individual differences in this hormonal variable. Thus, DHEAS met the statistical criteria for a biomarker of aging proposed above.

In addition, when comparing the slopes of age-related decline in adult males and females between humans and rhesus monkeys, the rate was about 2.3 times higher in monkeys, a rate that is consistent with humans' approximately three-fold greater lifespan. This evidence satisfied in part the fourth suggested criterion for a biomarker of aging, that species differences in the rate of age-related decline of the biomarker be proportional to the differences in their life spans.

In the NIA study, an initial analysis by Roth et al. (1993) following male monkeys after two to three years found no effects of CR on DHEAS levels. However, subsequent analysis after three to six years of CR revealed that the post-maturational decline in serum DHEAS was significantly attenuated in adult CR monkeys compared to controls (Lane et al. 1997). This result provided evidence for the beneficial effects of CR in postponing an age-related decline in hormonal function. Further analysis of this issue was required because of the circadian rhythmicity of DHEAS release. Thus, studies providing 24-hr sampling for hormonal levels are currently being conducted at the ONPRC. A preliminary analysis involving a small number of young adult (~ 10 years) and old male monkeys (~25 years) that had been on CR for about four years has been reported (Urbanski et al. 2004). In both diet groups, there was a significant age-related decline in mean and maximum plasma DHEAS concentrations that was not altered by CR. Interestingly, all young adult monkeys show a pronounced diurnal pattern that is nearly absent in the old monkeys. No significant difference in serum DHEAS between young CR and controls was found, but the levels in old CR monkeys were significantly lower compared to controls. Further studies using this procedure are being conducted in monkeys of different ages and sexes.

Melatonin is another potential hormonal biomarker of aging. Melatonin is secreted by the pineal gland and several other tissues, including the gastrointestinal tract, in a pulsatile pattern that peaks in the early morning (Klein et al. 1992). Melatonin has been reported to have many physiological effects, including involvement with sleep patterns, blood pressure, the immune system, and oxidative stress (Chase and Gidal 199; Skene et al. 1999; Anisimov et al. 1998; Nishiyama et al. 2001; Reiter 1995). The pineal gland shrinks with advancing age, associated with decreased melatonin secretion that can be accompanied by a shift in the phase of its pulsatile release (Nishiyama et al. 2001; Kripke et al. 1998). In contrast, melatonin secretion from the gastrointestinal tract can increase when calories are restricted.

In a cross-sectional study of NIA control monkeys, Roth et al. (2001) reported an age-related decline in peak melatonin levels in samples collected at night. Interestingly, a significant age-related decline was not evident in the young monkeys that had been maintained on CR for a 12-year period (Fig. 10 in Roth et al. 2001). However, melatonin levels in old CR monkeys (20–35 years) were significantly greater than those observed in the age-matched controls. Findings of sustained pineal function into old age in CR monkeys are consistent with those in CR rats (Stokkan et al. 1991) and suggest beneficial effects of CR in retarding this hormonal change. The finding that CR did not alter melatonin secretion in adult animals was not surprising, as they likely have not experienced significant age-related loss of this hormone. Similarly, a CR effect on melatonin levels was not observed among adult monkeys in the WNPRC (Ramsey et al. 2000). Diet differences may emerge as the monkeys are evaluated at older ages and assays are conducted using more reliable 24-hr sampling procedures available at the ONRPRC.

Products of glycation and glycoxidation have also been examined as biomarkers of aging (Sell et al. 2003). Products that can be measured in skin as a function of age, such as pentosidine and furosine, have been shown to increase with age in a variety of species, with the rate of change proportional to differences in life spans (Sell et al. 1996). Moreover, the age-related increase in their production in rodents has been reported to be attenuated by CR (Cefalu et al. 1995). Pentosidine and furosine showed positive correlations with age in rhesus CON monkeys in the NIA study but not in the CR groups. Moreover, the level of furosine as a measure of glycation was significantly lower among the aged group of monkeys (>20 years). As production of these products appears to accelerate in advanced age for the species studied to date, follow-up analysis among the group of older monkeys in the NIA study could prove insightful.

## Mortality and Morbidity

Some older monkeys in the NIA study have been on CR for over 17 years. The shortest time on CR is 12 years for some of the females. The current mortality rate is around 50% for aged monkeys begun in the study at ages ranging from 15–23 years. The current mortality rate for old CON monkeys is 50%, and the mortality rate for old CR monkeys is exactly the same. Thus, at this stage, there is no conclusion that CR is beneficial or detrimental to survival of older rhesus monkeys.

The leading cause of death in older monkeys is cancer. Again, the incidence of this disease among CON and CR monkeys is similar: 22% vs. 25%, respectively. Other causes of death among the old monkeys are cardiovascular disease, complications due to endometriosis, pneumonia, and liver failure, but the numbers of animals in each category are small and thus do not yet indicate any major differences in disease incidence between CON and CR monkeys.

## Summary and Conclusions

CR remains the only intervention demonstrated to consistently extend life span, reduce morbidity, and slow the rate of aging in short-lived animals. Rhesus monkeys exhibit many beneficial effects associated with CR that resemble those observed in CR rodents, such as decreased fat, improved glucoregulatory function, and decreased risk factors for cardiovascular disease and diabetes. Systematic studies of the effects of CR on older individuals from long-lived species have not been conducted to date. The NIA study of aging in rhesus monkeys offers this opportunity. Studies completed thus far indicate that older monkeys can respond to a 30% CR in a manner similar to young animals. For some variables, such as loss of fat, they do not respond as well. For other variables, such as increased production of melatonin, they apparently respond more robustly than young monkeys. Analysis of mortality and morbidity to date do not indicate any beneficial or detrimental effects of this nutritional regimen. Some variables, such as bone density, will need to be monitored closely to determine whether CR will have detrimental effects on aging. This study will continue to offer many new opportunities for assessing the effects of this nutritional intervention on aging processes in older nonhuman primates. In addition, further examination of the pattern of individual aging among the older cohorts of monkeys will permit characterization of frailty and underlying factors that predispose monkeys to this condition.

## Acknowledgments

The authors wish to acknowledge the valuable assistance of the staff at Poolesville, MD, including Edward Tilmont, April Hobbs, Jennifer Young, Tommy Thompson, Karl Reinsfelder, Alphie Ciser, and the veterinary staff, Drs. Doug Powell and Rick Herbert, as well as the support of Kris Rozankowski, our laboratory manager, at the Gerontology Research Center in Baltimore, MD. In addition, we acknowledge the abundant contributions of the many collaborators on this project at other research institutions.

## References

Anisimov VN, Mylnikov SV, Khavinson VK (1998) Pineal peptide preparation epithalamin increases the lifespan of fruit flies, mice, and rats. Mech Ageing Dev 1033:123–132

Barrett-Connor E, Khaw K, Yen S (1986) A prospective study of dehydroepiandrosterone sulfate, mortality, and cardiovascular disease. New Engl J Med. 315:1519–1524

Black A, Lane MA (2002) Nonhuman primate models of skeletal and reproductive aging. Gerontology 48:72–80

Black A, Allison DB, Shapses SA, Tilmont EM, Handy AM, Ingram DK, Roth GS, Lane MA (2001) Calorie restriction and skeletal mass in rhesus monkeys (Macaca mulatta): Evidence for an effect mediated through changes in body size. J Gerontol 56A:B98–B107

Bongaarts J (1980) Does malnutrition affect fecundity? A summary of evidence. Science 208: 564–569

Cefalu WT, Bell-Farrow AD, Wang ZQ, Sonntag WE, Fu MX, Baynes J, Thorpe SR (1995) Caloric restriction decreases age-dependent accumulation of the glycoxidation products, N epsilon-(carboxymethyl) lysine and pentodisine, in rat skin collagen. J Gerontol 50:BG337–341

Chase JE, Gidal BE (1997) Melatonin: therapeutic use in sleep disorders. Ann Pharmacother 10: 1218–1226

Colman R, Kemnitz JW (1998) Aging experiments using nonhuman primates. In: Yu BP (ed) Methods in aging research. Boca Raton: CRC Press. pp 249–267

Cutler RG, Davis BJ, Ingram DK, Roth GS (1992) Plasma concentrations of glucose, insulin, and percent glycated hemoglobin are unaltered by food restriction in rhesus and squirrel monkeys. J Gerontol 47:B9–B12

Dhahbi JM, Kim HJ, Mote PL, Beaver RJ, Spindler SR (2004) Temporal linkage between the phenotypic and genomic responses to caloric restriction. Proc Natl Acad Sci USA 101:5524–5529

De Laet CE, Van Hout BA, Burger H, Weel AE, Hofman A, Pols HA (1998) Hip fracture prediction in elderly men and women; validation in the Rotterdam study. J Bone Miner Res 13: 1587–1593

Edwards IJ, Rudel LL, Terry JG, Kemnitz JW, Weindruch R, Cefalu WT (1998) Caloric restriction in rhesus monkeys reduces low density lipoprotein interaction with arterial proteoglycans. J Gerontol 53A:B443–B448

Ensrud KE, Lipschutz RC, Cauley JA, Seeley D, Nevitt MC, Scott J, Orwoll ES, Genant HK, Cummings SR (1997) Body size and hip fracture risk in older women: a prospective study. Study of Osteoporotic Fractures Research Group. Am J Med 103:274–280

Fontana L, Meyer TE, Klein S, Holloszy JO (2004) Long-term calorie restriction is highly effective in reducing the risk for atherosclerosis in humans. Proc Natl Acad Sci USA 101:6659–6663

Forster MJ, Morris P, Sohal RS (2003) Genotype and age influence the effect of caloric intake on mortality in mice. FASEB J 17:690–692

Gordon T (1993) Factors associated with serum alkaline phosphatase level. Arch Pathol Lab Med 117:187–190

Goodrick CL, Ingram DK, Reynolds MA, Freeman JR, Cider N (1990) Effects of intermittent feeding upon body weight and lifespan in inbred mice: Interaction of genotype and age. Mech Ageing Devel 55:69–87

Heilbronn LK, Ravussin E (2003) Calorie restriction and aging: review of the literature and implications for studies in humans. Am J Clin Nutr 78:361–369

Holehan AM, Merry BJ (1985) Modification of the oestrous cycle hormonal profile by dietary restriction. Mech Ageing Devel 32:63–76

Ingram DK, Cutler RG, Weindruch R, Renquist DM, Knapka JJ, April M, Belcher CT, Clark MA, Hatcherson CD, Marriott BM, Roth GS (1990) Dietary restriction and aging: The initiation of a primate study. J Gerontol 45:B148–B163

Ingram DK, Nakamura E, Smucny D, Roth GS, Lane MA (2001) Strategy for identifying biomarkers of aging in long-lived species. Exp Gerontol 36:1025–1034

Jones ML (1968) Longevity of primates in captivity. Intl Zoo Yrbk 8: 183–192

Kaler LW, Gliessman P, Hess DL, Hill J (1986) The androgen status of aging male rhesus macaques. Endocrinology 119:566–571

Kalu DN, Hardin RR, Cockerham R, Yu BP (1984a) Aging and dietary modulation of rat skeleton and parathyroid hormone. Endocrinology 115:1239–1247

Kalu DN, Hardin RR, Cockerham R, Yu BP Norling BK, Egan JW (1984b) Lifelong food restriction prevents senile osteoporosis and hyperparathyroidism in F344 rats. Mech Ageing Devel 26:103–112

Kemnitz JW, Weindruch R, Roecker EB, Crawford K, Kaufman PL, Ershler WB (1993) Dietary restriction of adult male rhesus monkeys: design, methodology, and preliminary findings from the first year of the study. J Gerontol 48:B17–26

Kemnitz JW, Roecker EB, Weindruch R, Olson DF, Baum ST, Bergman RN (1994) Dietary restriction increases insulin sensitivity and lowers blood glucose in rhesus monkeys. Am J Physiol 266:E540–547

Kemnitz JW, Roecker EB, Haffa AL, Pinheiro J, Kurzman I, Ramsey JJ, Mac Ewen E.G (2000) Serum dehydroepiandrosterone sulfate concentrations across the life span of laboratory-housed rhesus monkeys. J Med Primatol 29:330–337

Krishnan KR, MM Husain, WM McDonald, Doraiswamy PM, Figiel GS, Boyko OB, Ellinwood EH, Nemeroff CB (1990) In vivo stereological assessment of caudate volume in man: Effects of normal aging. Life Sci 47:1325–1329

Klein DC, Roseboom PH, Donohue SJ, Marrs FL (1992) Evolution of melatonin as a night signal-contribution from a primitive photosynthetic organism. Mol Cell Neurosci 3:181–183

Koizumi A, Wada Y, Tsukada M, Hasegawa J, Walford RL (1989) Low blood glucose levels and small islets of Langerhans in the pancreas of calorie-restricted mice. Age 2:93–96

Kripke DF, Elliot JA, Youngstedet SD, Smith JS (1998) Melatonin: marvel or marker? Ann Med 30:81–87

Lane MA, Ball SS, Ingram DK, Cutler RG, Engel J, Read V, Roth GS (1995) Diet restriction in rhesus monkeys lowers fasting and glucose-stimulated glucoregulatory end points. Am J Physiol 268:E941–E948

Lane MA, Ingram DK, Ball SS, Roth GS (1997) DHEAS: A biomarker of primate aging slowed by calorie restriction. J Clin Endo Metab 82:2093–2096

Lane MA, Black A, Ingram DK, Roth GS (1998) Calorie restriction in nonhuman primates: Implications for age-related disease risk. J Antiaging Med 1:315–326

Lane MA, Tilmont EM, DeAngelis, H, Handy AM, Ingram DK, Kemnitz JW, Baum ST, Roth GS (2000) Short-term calorie restriction improves disease-related markers in older male rhesus monkeys (Macaca mulatta). Mech Ageing Dev 112:185–196

Lane MA, Black A, Handy AM, Shapses SA, Tilmont EM, Kiefer TL, Ingram DK, Roth GS (2001) Energy restriction does not alter bone mineral metabolism or reproductive cycling and hormones in female rhesus monkeys. J Nutr 131:820–827

Lindsay R, Bush TL, Grady D, Speroff L, Lobo RA (1996) Therapeutic controversy: estrogen replacement in menopause. J Clin Endocrinol Metab 81:3829–3838

Leblhuber F, Windhager E, Steinpartz FX, Dienstl E, Reisecker F, Rittmannsberger H (1991) Dehydroepiandrosterone-sulfate(DHEAS)serum levels in normal aging and Alzheimer's disease (AD). Age Ageing 14:116–118

Mascarucci P, Taub D, Saccani S, Paloma MA, Dawson H, Roth GS, Ingram DK, Lane MA (2001) Age-related changes in cytokine production by leukocytes in rhesus monkeys. Aging: Clin Exp Res 13:85–94

Mascarucci P, Taub D, Saccani S, Paloma MA, Dawson H, Roth GS, Lane MA, Ingram DK (2002) Cytokine responses in young and old rhesus monkeys: Effect of caloric restriction. J Interferon Cytokine Res 22:565–571

Masoro EJ, Compton C, Yu BP, Bertrand HA (1983) Temporal and compositional dietary restrictions modulate age-related changes in serum lipids. J Nutr 113:880–892

Matochick JA, Cherfer SI, Lane MA, Woolf RI, Morris ED, Ingram DK, Roth GS, London ED (2000) Age-related decline in striatal volume in monkeys as measured by magnetic resonance imaging. Neurobiol Aging 21:591–598

Matochik J, Chefer S, Roth G, Lane M, Mattison J, London E, Ingram D ( 2004) Age-related decline in striatal volume in rhesus monkeys: Assessments of long-term calorie restriction. Neurobiol Aging 25:193–200

Mattison J, Black A, Huck J, Moscrip T, Handy A, Tilmont E, Roth GS, Lane MA, Ingram DK (2004) Age-related decline in caloric intake and motivation for food in rhesus monkeys, Neurobiol Aging, in press.

Masoro E (2000) Calorie restriction and aging: an update. Exp Gerontol 35:299–305

Merry BJ, Holehan AM (1981) Serum profiles of LH, FSH, testosterone and 5 alpha-DHT from 21 to 1000 days of age in ad libitum fed and dietary restricted rats. Exp Gerontol 16:431–444

Moscrip TD, Ingram DK, Lane MA, Roth GS, Weed JL (2000) Locomotor activity in female rhesus monkeys: Assessment of age and calorie restriction effects. J Gerontol 55:B373–B380

Morris ED, Chefer SI, Lane MA, Muzic Jr. RF, Wong DF, Dannals RF, Matochik JA, Bonab AA, Villemagne VL, Grant SJ, Ingram DK, Roth GS, London E.D (1999) Loss of D2 receptor binding with age in rhesus monkeys: Importance of correction for differences in striatal size. J Cereb Blood Flow Metabol 19:218–229

Murphy DGM, DeCarli C, Schapiro MB, Rapoport SI, Horwitz B (1992) Age-related differences in volumes of subcortical nuclei, brain matter, and cerebrospinal fluid in healthy men as measured with magnetic resonance imaging. Arch Neurol 49:839–845

Nakamura E, Lane MA, Roth GS, Cutler RG, Ingram DK (1994) Evaluating measures of hematology and blood chemistry in male rhesus monkeys as biomarkers of aging. Exp Gerontol 29:151–177

Nakamura E, Lane MA, Roth GS, Ingram DK (1998) A strategy for identifying biomarder of agin: Further evaluation of hematology and blood chemistry data from a caloric restriction study in rhesus monkeys. Exp Gerontol. 35: 421–443

Nishiyama K, Yasue H, Moriyama Y, Tsunoda R, Ogawa H, Yoshimura M, Kugiyama K (2001) Acute effects of melatonin administration on cardiovascular autonomic regulation in healthy men. Am Heart J 141:E9

Ohasi M, Kato KI, Nawata H, Ibayashi H (1986) Adrenocortical responsiveness to graded ACTH infusions in normal young men and elderly human subjects. Gerontology 32:43–51

Orentreich N, Brind J, Rizer R, Vogelman J (1984) Age and sex differences in serum dehydroepiandrosterone sulfate concentrations throughout adulthood. J Clin Endocrinol Metab 59:551–555

Orentreich N, Brind JL, Vogelman JH (1992) Long-term longitudinal measurements of plasma dehydroepiandrosterone sulfate in normal men. J Clin Endocrinol Metab 75:1002–1004

Pyle SI, Waterhouse, AM, Greulich WW (1971) A radiographic standard of reference for the growing hand and wrist. Mosby-Year Book, St. Louis, MO

Ramsey JJ, Colman RJ, Binkley NC, Christensen JD, Gresl TA, Kemnitz JW, Weindruch R (2000) Dietary restriction and aging in rhesus monkeys: The University of Wisconsin study. Exp Gerontol 35:1131–1149

Raz N, Torres IJ, Acker JD (1995) Age, gender, and hemispheric differences in human striatum: A quantitative review and new data from in vivo MRI morphometry. Neurobiol Learn Mem 63:133–142

Reaven EPD, Wright CE, Mouden R, Solomon H, Reaven GM (1983) Effect of age and diet on insulin secretion and insulin action in the rat. Diabetes 32:175–179

Reiter RJ (1995) The pineal gland and melatonin in relation to aging: a summary of the theories and of the data. Exp Gerontol 30:199–212

Roecker, EB, Kemnitz JW, Ershler WB, Weindruch R (1996) Reduced immune response in rhesus monkeys subjected to diet restriction. J Gerontol 51:B276–B279

Roth GS, Blackman MR, Ingram DK, Lane MA, Ball SS, Cutler RG (1993) Age-related changes in androgen levels of rhesus monkeys subjected to diet restriction. Endocrine J 1:227–234

Roth GS, Lesnikov V, Lesnikov M, Ingram DK, Lane MA (2001) Dietary caloric restriction prevents the age-related decline in plasma melatonin levels of rhesus monkeys. J Clin Endo Metab 86:3293–3295

Roth GS, Mattison JA, Lane MA, Ottinger MA, Chachich M, Ingram DK (2004) Aging in rhesus monkeys: relevance to human health interventions. Science 305: 1423–1426

Sanderson JP, Binkley N, Roecker EB, Champ JE, Pugh TD, Aspnes L, Weindruch R (1997) Influence of fat intake and caloric restriction on bone in aging male rats. J Gerontol 52:B20–B25

Schwartz SM, Kemnitz JW (1992) Age- and gender-related changes in body size, adiposity, and endocrine and metabolic parameters in free-ranging rhesus macaques. Am J Phys Anthro 89: 109–121

Sell DR, Lane MA, Johnson WA, Masoro EJ, Mock OB, Reiser KM, Fogarty JF, Cutler RG, Ingram DK, Roth GS, Monnier VM (1996) Longevity and the genetic determination of collagen glycoxidation kinetics in mammalian senescence. Proc Natl Acad Sci USA 93:485–490

Sell DR, Lane MA, Obrenovich M, Mattison J, Handy A, Ingram DK, Cutler R, Roth GS, Monnier VM (2003) The effect of dietary restriction on glycation and glycoxidation in skin collagen of nonhuman primates, J Gerontol 58A:508–516

Skene DJ, Lockley SW, Arendt J (1999) Use of melatonin in the treatment of phase shift and sleep disorders. Adv Exp Med Biol 467:79–84

Small M, Gray CE, Beastall GH, MacCuish AC (1989) Adrenal androgens and insulin-dependent diabetes mellitus. Diabetes Res 11:93–95

Stokkan KA, Reiter RJ, Nonaka KO, Lerchl A, Yu BP, Vaughan MK (1991) Food restriction retards aging of the pineal gland. Brain Res 545:66–72

Tenover JS (1997) Testosterone and the aging male. J Androl 18:103–106

Thomas G, Frenoy N, Legrain S, Sebag-Lanoe R, Baulieu EE, Debuire B (1994) Serum dehydroepiandrosterone sulfate levels as an individual marker. J Clin Endocrinol Metab 79: 1273–1276

Urbanski HF, Downs JL, Garyfallou VT, Mattison JA, Lane MA, Roth GS, Ingram DK (2004) Effect of caloric restriction on thc 24-Hour plasma DHEAS and cortisol profiles of young and old male rhesus macaques. Ann NY Acad Sci 1019:443–447

Vallejo E (1957) La dieta de hambre a dias alternos en la alimentacion de los viejos. La Prensa Med Argentina 2:119–120

Verdery RB, Walford RL (1998) Changes in plasma lipids and lipoproteins in humans during a 2-year period of dietary restriction in Biosphere 2. Arch Intern Med 158:900-906

Verdery RB, Ingram DK, Roth GS, Lane MA (1997) Caloric restriction increases $HDL_2$ levels in rhesus monkeys (Macaca mulatta). Am J Physiol 273:E714- E719

Walford RL, Harris SB, Gunion MW (1992) The calorically-restricted low fat, nutrient dense diet in Biosphere 2 significantly lowers blood glucose, total leukocyte count, cholesterol and blood pressure in humans. Proc Natl Acad Sci USA 89:11533-11537

Walford RL, Mock D, Verdery R, MacCallum T (2002) Calorie restriction in biosphere 2: alterations in physiologic, hematologic, hormonal, and biochemical parameters in humans restricted for a 2-year period. J Gerontol 57:B211-224

Wanagat J, Allison DB, Weindruch R (1999) Caloric intake and aging: mechanisms in rodents and a study in nonhuman primates. Toxicol Sci 52(2 Suppl):35-40

Wood DH (1991) Long-term mortality and cancer risk in irradiated rhesus monkeys. Rad Res 126:132-140

Weed JL, Lane MA, Roth GS, Speer D, Ingram DK (1997) Activity measures in rhesus monkeys on long-term calorie restriction. Physiol Behav 62:97-103

Weindruch R, Walford RL (1988) The retardation of aging and disease by dietary restriction. Springfield: Charles C. Thomas.

Weindruch R, Lane MA, Ingram DK, Ershler WB, Roth GS (1997) Dietary restriction in rhesus monkeys: Lymphopenia and reduced mitogen-induced proliferation in peripheral blood mononuclear cells. Aging: Clin Expes 9:304-308

Yu B.P (1994) Modulation of aging process by dietary restriction. Boca Raton: CRC Press

Zumoff B, Levin J, Rosenfeld RS, Markham M, Starin GW, Fukushima DK (1981) Abnormal 24-hr mean plasma concentrations of dehydroepiandrosterone and dehydroepiandrosterone sulfate in women with primary operable breast cancer. Cancer Res. 41:3360-3363

# Evolutionary Perspectives on Human Longevity and Frailty

*Douglas E. Crews*[1]

According to its most avid supporters, the dawn of evolutionary medicine occurred during the latter part of the 20$^{th}$ century (Williams and Nesse 1991). Since then, evolutionary or Darwinian medicine has emerged as a leading theoretical perspective in medical and public health research (Trevathan et al. 1999; Williams and Nesse 1991). Evolutionary models have been applied to chronic degenerative diseases (CDDs), nutritional and infectious diseases, senescence and longevity, pharmacological sensitivities, obesity, and even patterns of infant mortality (see Crews and Gerber 1994; Eaton et al. 1997; Gerber and Crews 1999, 2003). Applications of the Darwinian paradigm to many practical problems in medicine, public health, and health care policy have been slower to develop, and applications to trauma, occupational health, and age-related frailty have yet to be examined. My purpose here is to examine the evolutionary background to frailty and longevity in modern humans through the lens of Darwinian medicine. In this context, frailty is viewed as all of the detrimental, age-related alterations in physical capabilities and physiological function secondary to trauma, disease, or senescence that reduce an individual's physiological reserve capacity and ability to respond to environmental or internal stress, thereby increasing their probability of death (see also Crews 2003).

The view of evolutionary medicine suggests that human evolutionary biology and phylogenetic inertia jointly contribute to both human frailty and longevity. Humankind's current patterns of life history (LH) and longevity suggest that frailty is dependent upon pre-existing adaptations that reflect a suite of co-adapted primate LH traits. These LH traits appear to be expressed most completely in humans but are also found among non-human primates and hominin ancestors of modern humans (Crews 2003; Gerber and Crews 2003). To understand patterns of frailty among today's aging population, plan health care policies, design living spaces for the elderly worldwide, or intervene on the processes of frailty among long-lived humans, an evolutionary understanding of associations among frailty, stress responses, survival, and longevity is needed.

One of the first questions to be asked – what is meant by frailty? – was addressed in the previous paragraph. Frailty is both a condition or state of being and a process of functional loss producing a greater susceptibility to intrinsic and extrinsic causes of death. To understand how frailty is structured in mod-

[1] Department of Anthropology and School of Public Health, The Ohio State University, 244 Lord Hall, 124 W. 17th Ave., Columbus, OH 43210-1364, USA, E-mail: Crews.8@osu.edu

Carey et al.
Longevity and Frailty

ern populations, it is necessary to examine the phylogenetic origins of frailty in our lineage. One avenue toward this end is to examine possible avenues of frailty among our non-human primate kin. Another is to examine the fossil and skeletal remains of our ancient and recent evolutionary forbearers to determine if they tell us anything about longevity and frailty in past populations. Examination of the skeletal remains from prehistoric and historic populations for possible activity and occupational influences on indicators of frailty may also provide an indication of how the evolution of human culture and behavior altered associations between longevity and frailty over time. Finally, assessments of frailty, along with its causes and consequences, among modern traditional-living populations will illustrate how frailty and survival are associated with one another today.

## Non-human Primates

In natural and free-ranging settings, wild non-human primates show a variety of traumatic injuries and generally shorter life spans than are observed among their caged kin. Studies of the recovered bones of wild-living primates reveal a variety of healed traumatic fractures. Joints and articular surfaces tend to show multiple signs of wear, erosion, atrophy, degenerative joint disease (DJD), osteoarthritis, and osteopenia in both macaques and humans as they age (DeRousseau 1985a,b; Williams and Bowden 1984). For example, Nakai (2003) recently examined 107 skeletons of macaques killed while crop raiding in Nagano Prefecture, Japan, and found 80 healed fractures in 31 of the 52 males and 71 in 26 of the 55 females. Among males, most fractures were in the trunk, clavicle, scapula, vertebrae, ribs and hip and appeared to have occurred during adult life; among females, the hand and foot most often showed signs of healed fractures that seem to have occurred during childhood and late life (Nakai 2003). DJD was also common among aged individuals, but osteoarthritis was not. The frequency of such conditions suggests that free-ranging primates sustain a variety of injuries and damage to their skeletal structures that reduce mobility, increase frailty, and reduce longevity. However, many of these skeletal lesions also show signs of healing, and individuals appear to have survived multiple traumatic episodes.

Among Gombe chimpanzees, Jurmain (1989) recovered the skeletal remains of 11 "old" individuals for examination of pathological lesions. Ten of these showed identifiable lesions that appeared to be secondary to traumatic injuries. The majority of fractures were observed in those with the highest estimated ages, with falls and interpersonal violence apparently the most common causes of skeletal lesions (Jurmain 1989). Interestingly, signs of degenerative diseases were fewer than would be expected from studies on human samples: only 2 of the 186 synovial joints and none of the 344 intervertebral joints showed any signs of DJD (Jurmain 1989). In addition, Jurmain (1989) reported a complete lack of osteophytosis, in contrast to what is common among older humans. All large-bodied primates appear to show less osteoarthritis, osteoporosis and DJD, particularly of the spine, than do humans; in addition, the major peripheral joints of apes show less DJD (Jurmain 2000). The low prevalence of DJD among wild-living large-bodied apes also differs from what is observed among macaques and other small-bodied Catherine primates reared in captivity (Jurmain 2000). Such data suggest that the human bipedal gait is achieved at great biomechanical costs, leading to ubiquitous vertebral changes and lower back pain by the fifth decade in humans (see Jurmain 1989, 2000). They also suggest that human patterns of frailty may be quite different, at least with respect to skeletal degeneration, from those of our closest ape relatives. Caged primates tend to show a different suite of bone lesions and losses than do the free-living (DeRousseau et al. 1987). Different habitual activity patterns within different size enclosures also appear to produce differential skeletal stress and variable patterns of bone loss in caged versus free-ranging non-human primates (see also Turnquist 1983).

## Hominin and Human Ancestors

Although the fossil record of hominin evolution is patchy and relatively few specimens are available for study, our Australopithecine and Erectine forbearers likely experienced a variety of fractures, parasitic conditions, and osteoarthritic conditions similar to those observed among modern large-bodied apes and later Neanderthals, for whom more evidence is available. Evidence of trauma and the possibility of associated frailty are more clearly identifiable among Neanderthal remains than among those of earlier hominins (Trinkhaus and Zimmerman 1982; Zollikofer et al. 2002). For example, among the Shanidar Neanderthals, four showed clear evidence of healed antemortem trauma (Trinkhaus and Zimmerman 1982). The Shanidar 1 specimen exhibits healed trauma and subsequent hypoplasia of the right shoulder area, along with DJD of the right knee, ankle, and foot. Shanidar 3 also shows DJD of the right foot, in association with a penetrating wound to the ninth rib, whereas specimen 4 exhibits a healed fracture of a rib and Shanidar 5 a healed wound to the left frontal bone (Trinkhaus and Zimmerman 1982). The wound to specimen 3's rib and the wound to the left frontal bone of specimen 5 (possibly due to a blow to the head from a right-handed adversary), and the fractured rib suggest that interpersonal violence may have been their cause. Such findings suggest that interpersonal violence, accidental trauma, and post-trauma survival were frequent among Neanderthals (Berger and Trinkhaus 1995; Trinkhaus and Zimmerman 1982). This high survival rate post-trauma also suggests that a supportive social setting that provided the opportunity for provisioning of disabled individuals was in place among Neanderthals.

A wide variety of skeletal and dental aberrations also characterized our more recent ancestors. Some of these appear to have been secondary to habitual activities that produced unusual postures; others were due to the habitual use of the limbs and dentition as tools (see Kennedy 1989; Wilczak and Kennedy 1998). Stress on either muscle, teeth, or bone may leave marks on skeletal elements. Dental attrition may reflect use of the teeth in processing wood tools and leather or a coarse diet throughout life. Both rapid dental formation during youth or early dental attrition may reflect a diet of coarse and abrasive foodstuffs. This may have been the case for some Neanderthals whose dental remains show early and rapid eruption and rapid wear (Thompson and Nelson 2000). The Neanderthal pattern of growth and development does not fit that of either modern gorillas or humans or that of earlier Erectines (Thompson and Nelson 2000). Early development of Neanderthal dentition may have resulted to accommodate their poorer nutritional base, coarser diet, and lower levels of parental investment (PI) as compared to contemporary *Homo sapiens sapiens* (see Crews 2003). These data further suggest that Neanderthals may not have had as great an opportunity during their growth period to develop the physiological organ reserves (a specific type of frailty) that allow modern humans to experience late-life survival. The longer growth period of modern humans allows them to establish a greater reserve capacity that ultimately can be converted into longer-term survival (Crews 2003).

A number of human cultural activities that leave their marks on bone may also have contributed to increased frailty among earlier humans and may still do so among modern ones. Carrying of burdens on the head or the use of line cords for hauling activities may result in fractures of the cervical vertebrae and subsequent loss of function and constant pain (see Kennedy 1989). Spear throwing, along with sword and sling usage, may result in hypertrophy of the proximal ulna due to hyperextension of the arm (see Kennedy 1989), a condition that may appear particularly frequently in medieval cemetery materials. Bone degeneration, osteoporosis, and osteoarthritis are all accelerated among the obese and those who practice heavy physical labor on a regular basis, and they contribute to increased individual frailty with increasing age. Many of these conditions have been identified and aggregated as markers of occupational stress (MOS) by Kennedy (1989) and his colleagues (Wilczak and Kennedy 1998). The "osteological paradox" suggests that skeletal materials exhibiting the greatest number or amount of traumatic lesions are likely to represent the most physically fit and longest-lived individuals in their population. This is because they were the ones who survived these stresses, whereas those who failed to survive are represented by skeletons with few or no signs of lesions, because they died following their traumatic or illness episode. Thus, those who survived into later ages may have had the most frailty but also the greatest recuperative abilities.

At least one modern sample suggests that this may still be the case among foraging and horticultural populations. Sugiyama (2004) investigated 673 injuries among a sample of 40 Shiwiar forager-horticulturalists living in Ecuadorian Amazonia. He reported that injury and illness were major aspects of life, occurring often across the life span and frequently leading to temporary disabilities that were sufficiently severe to have been life threatening without provisioning of food and resources by others in the population. The fitness effects associated with such provisioning were extrapolated to be significantly high to influence reproductive success and life span, since young adults were often affected (Sugiyama 2004). Provisioning effectively lowered mortality in this small-scale society, thereby allowing multiple members to survive periods of high disability that could cause or eventually lead to increased frailty. Extrapolating from living populations to those of past millennia is always fraught with problems; however, these observations among the Shiwiar, along with multiple additional lines of evidence (see Crews 2003) suggest that one of the major adaptive strategies that humans have followed is group cooperation leading to behaviors such as provisioning. Provisioning as part of the human biocultural adaptive suite sets latter hominins apart from their modern ape relatives and pre-human ancestors. Provisioning along with high PI during growth and development, and for decades beyond attainment of maximum reproductive potential, are human adaptations that not only set us apart but also contribute to a disconnection between frailty and mortality/longevity in our species (see Crews 2003).

## Frailty Among Modern Humans

Patterns of frailty today vary widely across the world's many and varied populations. For example, the Shiwiar of the Ecuadorian Amazon experience quite different risks of disability and illness than do we in our more cosmopolitan settings. Similarly, those living in the slums of Calcutta and Mexico City are exposed to very different stressors, injuries, and diseases than are citizens of London, New York, or Paris. Yet, the likelihood that they, you, or I will experience some loss of physiological function or physical capability as we age is quite real. Those living in the slums of Calcutta may experience death (a permanent type of disability/frailty) before they lose physiological function and well before someone residing in a more cosmopolitan setting may experience disability or frailty, but frailty is always a possibility.

How disability or frailty is assessed also in part determines whom we classify as frail or not. In the US, the most commonly reported assessment of disability and frailty is one's self-report of their ability to complete activities of daily living (ADLs; Katz et al. 1963). This measurement scale is based upon one's ability to complete tasks such as bathing, dressing, transferring (moving from a chair to bed or the toilet and vice versa), toileting, ambulating, and feeding oneself (Katz et al. 1963). In vogue since their development in the early 1960s, ADLs have been assessed on a broad spectrum of samples both young and old. The scale items also have been included in a number of representative cross-sectional surveys of US citizens. Over time, the proportions reporting loss of ability to complete at least one ADL by age cohort have generally declined. For example, in a 1984 representative sample of US elders, among those aged 65–74 years of age, 15% of men and 18% of women reported that they could not complete at least one ADL without aid. Among those aged 75–84, 20% and 31% of men and women, respectively, reported they could not, and among those 85+, 40% and 53% (NCHS 1987, Brook et al. 1990). In a 1987 representative survey, only 5% and 6.5% of 65-to 69-year-old US men and women, respectively, reported that they had difficulty with at least one ADL, while among those 85+, 26% and 38% did (Rakowski and Pearlman 1995). At about the same time, the rate of self-reported disability among US citizens aged 65+ also apparently declined from about 24.9% in 1982 to 21.3% in 1994 ($p<0.0001$; Manton et al. 1997). Data from such large representative surveys in cosmopolitan settings suggest that frailty is lower among older cohorts today than it was among the same age cohorts in previous decades. That is, we are healthier, more active, and less frail today than were our grandparents at the same ages.

Frailty due to trauma, disease, "bad genes" and interpersonal violence always has been an inherent aspect of hominin and human existence. However, two socioculturally related trends, extended PI in offspring and provisioning by others in the social group during periods of disability, along with technological improvements appear to have lessened the severity of these contributors to frailty. During the latter part of the 20th century, in more cosmopolitan populations, morbidity from chronic degenerative diseases commonly associated with aging, senescence and increased frailty was pushed to older ages, such that those aged 65–74 now experience a rate similar to what those aged 55–64 experienced early in the 20th century (Crews 2003). Even among the oldest-old, mortality rates declined steadily during the latter half of the 20th century, as seen, for example, among those 100+ years of age in Japan (Robine 2003) and Holland (Wilmoth 1998). Longevity appears to have been decoupled, to some extent, from the dual scourges of CDDs and frailty, at least in the most well-off segments of cosmopolitan societies.

A new model for assessing relationships between longevity and frailty may be allostatic load. Introduced to the gerontological and health care literature by Bruce McEwen (1998, 2000), Theresa Seeman, and colleagues (1997, 2001), allostatic load is a composite of multiple measures of physiological function that respond to psychosocial and physiological stressors. As defined by these researchers, allostatic load is based on 10 physiological factors; others have used as few as seven or as many as 23. Following McEwen (1998), the components of allostatic load include systolic and diastolic blood pressure, waist/hip ratio, HDl- and total-cholesterol, glycated hemoglobin, serum dihydroepiadosterone, and overnight urinary cortisol, adrenaline, and noradrenaline. Allostatic load is scored as the sum of physiological measures in the highest quartile of risk. Measured thus, allostatic load is associated with mortality and cognitive and functional declines among elderly participants in the MacArthur Studies of Successful Aging (Karlamangla et al. 2002; Seeman et al.. 2001) and days of work missed by middle-aged men (Johnston-Brooks et al. 1998). Allostatic load appears to be higher at older ages across current US cohorts through the seventh decade of life but stable thereafter; it is also associated with selective mortality in this representative sample of the US population (Crimmins et al. 2003). Crimmins et al. (2003) suggest that allostatic load may increase with increasing age in the US and that its stability after age 60 reflects selective the mortality of those with the highest scores. In at least one non-US sample, American Samoa, allostatic load shows a negative association with age in a culture with a very different population history and life ways than observed in the US (Crews 2003).

Another scale being developed specifically to assess physical frailty is the Clinical Global Impression of Change in Physical Frailty (CGIC-PF) instrument (Studenski et al. 2004). This consensus-based scale includes both quantitative and qualitative items, was developed by a team of clinicians, patients, caregivers, and other "experts," and shows a reliability estimate of 0.97 (Studenski et al. 2004). The CGIC-PF covers six intrinsic domains, including mobility, endurance, balance, nutrition, strength, and neuromotor performance, and seven consequence domains: medical complexity, health care use, appearance, ADLs, self-perceived health, and emotional and health status. Change in any domain is scored on a scale of 1–7, with 1 indicating markedly worse, 4 no change, and 7 markedly improved (Studenski et al. 2004). An advantage of both the allostatic load and CGIC-PF assessments is that they are expected to change over time for any one individual, just as frailty changes over time, and change can be used to gauge an individual's trajectory.

## Discussion

Longevity and frailty are permanently linked in the minds of the public, physicians, and gerontological researchers. These linkages are based on historical and evolutionary patterns that showed that as one aged one also lost physiological functions and became increasingly frail. However, current data suggest that this is not necessarily the case today, and it may not have been true even in the recent past. In fact, data from modern representative samples suggest that: 1) morbidity and mortality rates from the CDDs commonly associated with increasing age are declining across the life span, and 2) loss of ability to perform ADLs, an indicator of frailty, also is lower among currently aging cohorts than it was in earlier cohorts at the same ages. However, even though frailty and longevity may be becoming disconnected to some degree, among those dying at ages over 80, all organ systems (with the exception of the liver) show progressive pathology, suggesting that a system-wide loss of function still increases with age in cosmopolitan settings (see Carnes et al. 2003). What this all may suggest is that frailty, a manifestation of functional loss, is declining among cohorts at older ages compared to their grandparents because the conditions that promote frailty are being slowed. However, the pathological processes that ultimately lead to death are continuing, albeit at a slower pace than in previous generations and with fewer obvious losses, throughout the latter years. These processes are today being held in abeyance across many more decades of life than ever before by medical technology, pharmacology, nutritional improvements, and healthier life styles, leading to prolonged life with fewer disabilities for many. Thus, among the oldest-old, multiple competing conditions contribute to death, suggesting that the underlying cause of death may be loss of reserve capacity, frailty, and just plain old age, an underlying cause of death that has been eliminated from our most recent International Classifications of Diseases, Illnesses and Causes of Death.

## References

Berger TD, E. Trinkaus (1995) Patterns of trauma among Neandertals. J Archaeol Sci 22: 841–852.

Brook DB, Guralnik JM, Brody JA (1990) Demography amd epidemiology of aging in the United States. In: Schneider EL, Rose JW (eds) Handbook of the biology of aging. San Diego: Academic Press, Inc. pp 3–23.

Carnes BA, Olshansky SJ, Grahn D (2003) Biological evidence for limits to the duration of life. Biogerontology 4:31–45.

Gerber LM, Crews DE (1999) Evolutionary perspectives on chronic degenerative diseases. In: Trevathin W, Mckenna J, Smith N (eds) Evolutionary medicine. New York: Oxford University Press, pp. 443–69.

Crews DE (2003) Human senescence: evolutionary and biocultural perspectives. Cambridge: Cambridge University Press.

Crews DE, Gerber LM (1994) Chronic degeneratice diseases and aging. In: Crews DE, Garruto (eds) Biological anthropology and aging: perspectives on human variation over the life span. New York, Oxford University Press, pp. 174–208.

Crimmins EM, Johnston M, Hayward M, Seeman T (2003) Age differences in allostatic load: an index of physiological dysregulation. Exp Gerontol 38:731–734.

DeRousseau CJ (1985a) Aging in the musculoskeletal system of Rhesus monkeys: III. Degenerative joint disease. Am J Phys Anthropol 68:177–184.

DeRousseau CJ (1985b) Aging in the musculoskeletal system of Rhesus monkeys: III. Bone loss. Am J Phys Anthropol 68:157–167.

DeRousseau CJ, Bito LZ, Kaufman PL (1987) Aging and life cycles in non-human primates. Paper presented at the 40th Annual Scientific Meeting of the Gerontological Society of America. The Gerontol 27 (Special Issue): 12.

Eaton SB, Eaton III SB, Konner MJ (1997) Paleolithic nutrition revisited: A twelve-year retrospective on its nature and implications. Eur J Clin Nutr 51:207–216.

Gerber LM, Crews DE (2003) Chronic degenerative diseases and human evolution. In: Canali S, Carbellini G (eds) Medicinia Darwiniana L'Approccio Evoluzionista alla Malattia. Apeiron Editora Comunicazione SRL: Italy

Johnston-Brooks CH, Lewis MA, Evans GW, Whalen CK (1998) Chronic stress and illness in children: the role of allostatic load. Psychosomat Med 60:597–603.

Jurmain R (1989) Trauma, degenerative disease, and other pathologies among the Gombe chimpanzees. Am J Phys Anthropol 80:229–237.

Jurmain R. (2000) Degenerative joint disease in African great apes: an evolutionary perspective. J Human Evol 39(2): 185–203.

Karlamangla AS, Singer BH, McEwen BS, Rowe JW, Seeman TE (2002) Allostatic load as a predictor of functional decline: MacArthur studies of successful aging. J Clin Epidemiol 55:696–710.

Katz SA, Ford AB, Moskowitz RW, Jackson BA, Jaffee MW (1963) Studies of illness in the aged. The index of ADL: a standardized measure of biological and psychosocial function. JAMA 185:914–919.

Kennedy KAR (1989) Skeletal markers of occupational success. In: Iscan MY, Kennedy KAR (eds) Reconstruction of life from the skeleton. New York: Liss Inc., pp. 129–160.

Manton KG, Corder L, Stallard E (1997) Chronic disability trends in elderly United States populations: 1982–1994. Proc Natl Acad Sci USA 94: 2593–2598.

McEwen BS (1998) Protective and damaging effects of stress mediators. New Engl J Med 338:171–179.

McEwen BS (2000) The neurobiology of stress: from serendipity to clinical relevance. Brain Res 2000; 886: 172–89.

Nakai, M (2003) Bone and joint disorders in wild Japanese macaques from Nagano Prefecture, Japan. Intl J Primatol 24: 179–195.

Rakowski W, Pearlman DN (1995) Demographic aspects of aging: current and future trends. In: Reicher W (ed) Care of the elderly: clinical aspects of aging. Baltimore: Williams and Wilkins, pp. 488–495.

Robine JM, Yasuhiko S, Jagger C (2003) The emergence of extremely old people: the case of Japan. Exp Gerontol 38:735–739.

Seeman TE, Singer BH, Rowe JW Horwitz RI, McEwen BS (1997) The price of adaptation – allostatic load and its health consequences: MacArthur studies of successful aging. Arch Intern Med 157: 2259–2268.

Seeman TE, McEwen BS, Rowe JW, Singer BH (2001) Allostatic load as a marker of cumulative biological risk: MacArthur studies of successful aging. Proc Natl Acad Sci USA 98: 4770–4775.

Studenski S, Hayes RP, Leibowitz RQ, Bode R, Lavery L, Walston J, Duncan P, Perera S (2004) Clinical global impression of change in physical frailty: development of a measure based on clinical judgement. J Am Ger Soc 52:1560–1566.

Sugiyama LS.(2004) Illness, injury, and disability among Shiwiar forager-horticulturalists: implications of health-risk buffering for the evolution of human life history. Am J Phys Anthropol 123:371–389.

Sugiyama Y (2004) Demographic parameters and life history of chimpanzees at Bossou Guinea. Am J Phys Anthropol 124:154–165.

Thompson JL Nelson AJ (2000) The place of Neanderthals in the evolution of hominid patterns of growth and development. J Human Evol 38:475–495.

Trankhaus E, Zimmerman MR (1982) Trauma among the Shanidar Neandertals. Am J Phys Anthropol 57:61–76

Trevathan WR, McKenna JJ, Smith N (1999) Evolutionary medicine. Oxford University Press: New York, pp. 443–469.

Turnquist JE (1983) Caging and joint mobility. Am J Phys Anthropol 60:263

Williams DD, Bowden DM (1984) A nonhuman primate model for the osteopensia of aging. In: Scarpelli DG, Migaki G (eds) Comparative pathobiology of major age-related diseases. New York: Alan R. Liss. 207–220

Williams GC, Nesse RM (1991) The dawn of Darwinian medicine. Quart Rev Biol 66:1–22.

Wilmoth JR (1998) The future of human longevity: a demographer's perspective. Science 280: 395–397

Wilzack C, Kennedy K (1998) Mostly Mos: technical aspects of identification of skeletal markers of occupational stress. In: Reichs KJ (ed) Forensic osteology: advances in the identification of human remains Springfield: Charles C Thomas, pp 461–490

Zollikofer CPE, de Leon MSP, Vandermeersch B, Leveque F (2002) Evidence for interpersonal violence in the St. Cesaire Neanderthal. Proc Natl Acad Sci USA 99: 6444–6448.

# Flies Without Wings

*Lois M. Verbrugge*[1]

## Introduction

In demography and public health sciences, frailty has become a prominent topic of aging research, joining the longstanding interest in mortality. By comparison, frailty has had little role in biological research on animal models of aging; mortality is the preeminent outcome of interest. We discuss how demography and biology can interact in fruitful ways, so that frailty is considered for inclusion in animal models. If this occurs, animal models will have stronger implications for human aging, where both quantity and quality of life are paramount concerns.

The title "Flies Without Wings" derives from a conference of demographers and biologists in the late 1980's. An evolutionary biologist presented work on long-lived *drosophila* flies. A demographer asked what the very old flies looked like. "Oh, their wings fall off," the biologist replied in cavalier manner. This astonished the demographers. Experimental models for flies had achieved longevity without attention to late-life function? What then was their genuine relevance for human aging? Policies and therapies that increase humans' length of life but entail profound disability (analogous to wings falling off) would be unacceptable in human society. I promptly wrote "Flies Without Wings" on a piece of paper, as a fine title for a manuscript about the disjunction in research on human aging versus other animals. It is a key theme of this paper.

## The concept of frailty in demography and public health sciences

We begin with the transition in recent decades from evocative description of frailty to its careful measurement in demography and public health sciences.

[1] Asia Research Institute, Shaw Foundation Bldg. (Block AS7, Level 4), 5 Arts Link, National University of Singapore, Singapore 117570; (65) 6874 5243 (tel), (65) 6779 1428 (fax); arivlm@nus.edu.sg (email); *from 09/05*: Lois M. Verbrugge, Institute of Gerontology, 300 North Ingalls, University of Michigan, USA 48109-2007; (1) 734-936-2103 (tel); (1) 734-936-2116 (fax); verbrugg@umich.edu (email)

Carey et al.
Longevity and Frailty

## Descriptions and their Transit to Science

Frailty is a common word in lay speech, and its colloquial meaning is clear. When a friend says, "My mother is frail," the mother's status is unambiguous. She is physically fragile, vulnerable to accidents, and could die at any time.

Professionals in geriatrics, nursing, demography, and public health sciences have provided simple descriptions of frailty in professional terms: reduced physiological reserves, vulnerability to adverse outcomes, loss of physiological complexity, inability to compensate, unstable homeostasis, wasting, lack of robustness, low resilience, sub-clinical conditions, failure of redundancy (e.g., Bennett, 2004; Felten and Hall, 2001; Roubenoff, 1999). Professionals view frailty as a syndrome involving multiple body systems (Ferrucci et al. 2003). Most often cited as components are musculoskeletal, neuroendocrine, nutritional, and immunological/inflammation systems (Fried and Walston, 1999; Kinney, 2004; Morley et al. 2002; Walston, 2004). Several articles discuss the notion of multisystem failure in theoretical ways (Bortz, 1993; Lipsitz, 2002, 2004), and others discuss frailty within its broader social, psychological, and cultural spheres (Baltes and Smith, 2003; Raphael et al. 1995; Robine and Michel, 2004; Schulz and Williamson, 1993). As research interest in frailty has risen, good reviews of the concept have been written (Fried et al. 2004; Hamerman, 1999; Hogan et al. 2003; Kinney, 2004, Markle-Reid and Browne, 2003; Rockwood et al. 2000; Wells et al. 2003). Most discuss how frailty is a distinctive phenomenon, different from aging and disability. Several conference reports and calls for grant proposals also review the concept (Hadley et al. 1993; National Institute on Aging, 2003; National Institutes of Health, 1991).

## Frailty and Impairments

Descriptions of frailty in lay and professional language are evocative, and they serve as inspiration for science. A hallmark of science is measurement, and scientists have worked to transform the concept of frailty into indicators for empirical research. A good starting point for this effort is the specific features of frailty stated by clinicians, such as rapid unintended weight loss, persistent or easy fatigue, unsteady gait, weakness, disinterest in milieu, physically inactive, poor appetite, impaired cognition, depression (e.g., Bales and Ritchie, 2002; Cohen, 2000; Morley, 2001; Muhlberg and Sieber, 2004). Clinicians typically describe a set of features whose coexistence indicates frailty.

Frailty fits neatly and easily into the basic architecture of the disablement process (Verbrugge and Jette, 1994). The disablement process presents a basic pathway from chronic and acute health problems to disability, as follows: pathology → impairments → functional limitations → disability. Briefly, pathology can prompt impairments in specific body systems; they in turn can cause limitations in basic functioning, and thence disability in whole activities of a person's life. An example pathway is osteoarthritis that causes limited range of motion, pain, and loss of muscle mass. These can cause difficulty walking, stooping, reaching, or climbing stairs, and a person may then have difficulty going to church, doing housework, and getting to his/her job. The disablement process is reciprocal since functional limitations and disability can exacerbate the health conditions and impairments that initiated them.

Frailty pertains to impairments. Impairments are dysfunctions or significant abnormalities in specific body systems (physical, sensory/communication, mental/emotional). This is a central arena for clinical evaluations of individuals. Simply described, impairments are "signs and symptoms." The features in the first paragraph are symptoms.

The distinction between impairments and functional limitations can be confusing because clinical evaluations are often a mélange of both. Impairments are physiological features and their immediate manifestations --signs and symptoms, respectively. An impairment is usually within a single body system (e.g., reduced range of motion, low visual acuity, low respiratory volume), or occasionally is a whole-body feature (e.g., fatigue, malaise). By contrast, functional limitations are difficulties a person has doing basic physical or mental behaviors (e.g., walking, speaking, paying attention). (These basic behaviors serve as building blocks for whole activities, e.g., going to work, talking with friends, learning. Difficulty doing whole tasks due to health is disability.)

## Complexities of Frailty

If the background above were sufficient, the task of measuring frailty would be quite simple: choose specific impairments, measurement procedures, and demarcation points that signify severe dysfunction for each impairment. But the frailty concept is more complex. First, frailty is a constellation of impairments, or a syndrome. Multiplicity is a central aspect. Is the syndrome a single well-defined set of impairments, or can there be various subsets within the full set? Are there interactions among particular impairments that signal frailty? Second, there may be a key system whose dysfunction unlocks the frailty process. This body system may be sufficient, or sufficient and necessary. The musculoskeletal system is often nominated as the key system (Bortz, 1993; Ferrucci, 2005; Marcell, 2003). Third, there may be limiting factors that occur during the frailty process. This notion derives from industrial engineering: for jobs with many component tasks, inability to do a particular one means the entire job cannot be accomplished. Translated to frailty, if dysfunction in a body system reaches a given level, other systems rapidly decline, and there is little chance for recovery. The idea of weak link is similar. Fourth, impairments are likely nonlinear with regard to frailty. Within a given body system, scores can descend or rise to some point without dire consequences and with good possibility for clinical intervention; the situation changes radically after that point. Summing up, frailty's complexity is appreciated by contemporary researchers (Ferrucci, 2005; Morley et al. 2002), but operationalizing that complexity is difficult.

## Empirical Measures of Frailty

What are some measures of frailty in contemporary research that focus on body system impairments?

The most common approach is to select sets of items from surveys or clinical evaluations, choose cutpoints that indicate low function for each item, add up how many low-function items a person has, and set a cutoff point for the sum to define the subgroup of frail persons (e.g., Binder et al. 2002; Fried et al. 2001; Mitnitski et al. 2001; 2004; Shlipak et al. 2004; some have item sets extending beyond impairments). Some studies count instead the number of body systems with low-function items; this approach accommodates the idea of multisystem presentation (Matthews et al. 2004; Strawbridge et al. 1998). Several empirical studies propose that just one or two indicators suffice as markers of frailty (Chin et al. 2003; Hardy and Gill, 2004; Syddall et al. 2003; others in Morley et al. 2002).

The content of item sets has changed a great deal in the past 15 years, and we provide a brief history. Initially, item sets were often potpourris that included both impairments and functional limitations. Gradually, more conceptual integrity has worked its way into research, and item sets now usually concentrate on symptoms. Symptom sets are relatively easy to obtain from physician reports or self-reports; they do not require laboratory-based measurements. Current work by Walston and colleagues is pushing back the frontier into the basic physiology of frailty (Ferrucci et al. 2002; Walston, 2005; Walston and Fried, 1999; Walston et al. 2002; see also Lamberts et al. 1997; Vanitallie, 2003). The items are biomarkers of frailty (signs), and they involve laboratory-based assessments. Attention is especially focused on inflammation, coagulation, endocrine, and metabolic features. The team's current goal is to identify signs that distinguish frail and nonfrail persons, previously defined by a well-evaluated symptom set.

Besides sets of impairment items, there are two other genuine types of frailty indicators. One is the presence of critical clinical indicators. Sarcopenia is most often nominated as an indicator of frailty (Marcell, 2003; Morley et al. 2001; Roubenoff, 2000). It is a syndrome more than a disease, and is often evaluated by a holistic clinical perspective. The second indicator is overall judgment by a professional, other caregiver, or the individual him/herself. This gestalt approach is simple and straightforward, yet rarely present in the literature (Matthews et al. 2004). Self-rated health is a gestalt measure, and demographers have learned its great value as a predictor of outcomes. That should prompt us to develop and assess gestalt measures of frailty.

## Inclusion

Can surveys obtain answers from frail people? For decades, standard survey practice has been to exclude eligible people who prove difficult to reach, and they become part of the nonresponse group. Further, exclusion can happen during study design. Whole categories of people who are relevant but deemed difficult to interview, are excluded from the sample. They are made ineligible for the study.

Frail people can be indeed be difficult to reach and interview because of their communication problems and gatekeepers. But the convenient assumptions that people in very poor health cannot provide information about themselves, and that it costs too much, must be dropped. Contemporary survey practice is rapidly changing to include tailored strategies to recruit and interview people with very compromised health and function. Interview procedures that are different, slower, and "client-focused" are successful in obtaining answers from many, even most, of them (Interagency Committee on Disability Research, 2004; see also Barron et al. 2004; Ferrucci et al. 2004 ).

## Checkpoints

Several general questions may aid researchers as they develop frailty indicators. First, do the candidate items measure frailty itself or, instead, its consequences (functional limitations, disability, death)? Second, would frailty be measured differently for children and youths than for elderly persons? Is the measurement protocol actually age-specific? If so, one can work to prepare a more age-inclusive protocol, or else simply acknowledge that the protocol pertains to older persons and its applicability to other age groups is unknown. Third, what is the opposite of frailty, and how would that be measured? For example, how is physiological homeostasis (multisystem balance) measured, or high resilience, or physiological redundancy? Ideally, we would like items and protocols that span best to worst status. This is feasible for some indicators, but quite intractable for many others. Fourth, is frailty a state or a process? It is likely best viewed as a process, and is ideally measured that way, as a trajectory of signs or symptoms. The first step is to develop sophisticated and conceptually clear protocols with one-time-point measurement, then extend these to over-time. Fifth, how do frailty and typical declines with aging differ? Do the chosen indicators reflect a distinctive status or, instead, something that often occurs as people get older? Professionals and scientists think frailty is distinctive, so protocols need to measure its specialness.

## Consequences of frailty

The consequences of frailty are the inability to perform activities and roles, need for personal assistance in daily activities, falls and other unintended injuries, high medical care expenses and hospital stays, residence changes such as institutionalization and hospice, early death relative to age peers, or death due to particular causes. There is research literature on frailty's link to these outcomes (e.g., Black and Rush, 2002; Covinsky et al. 2003; Fried et al. 2001; Gessert et al. 2002; Hardy and Gill, 2004; Imuta et al. 2001; Lunney et al. 2002; 2003; Manton, 1986; Matthews et al. 2004; Mehdizadeh, 2002; Mitnitski et al. 2002; 2004; Winograd et al. 1991).

I hypothesize that frailty's most distinctive consequences are functional trajectories, that is, the forms and speeds of functional change. Frailty is linked more strongly to functional trajectories than to types or degrees of functional limitations. This hypothesis is very general, comparing the relative importance of longitudinal dynamics and cross-sectional status. The real crux of the matter is: which specific forms and speeds of functional trajectory are most linked to frailty? My guess is that frailty causes unstable downward momentum to function. Unstable means high day-to-day, week-to-week variability. In observational terms, someone who cares for an elderly person cannot predict if tomorrow will be better, the same, or worse. The trajectory's overall speed may be slow, swift, or some combination, such as slow-then-swift. I make no guess on this, but suspect frailty has several indicative speed trajectories.

We greatly need measures of patterns and paces of change in function. Empirical heft for notions of "cascade," "lingering," "catastrophic decline," "instability," "downward spiral," "vicious cycle," and other functional trajectories described in the literature is weak or absent. To accomplish this requires not only longitudinal data, but innovative variables that represent fully each person's variation over time.

In a footnote, I summarize empirical work on disability patterns and changes in disability patterns.[1] There is little literature on patterns of functional limitations. The summary shows how researchers routinely condense data for ease of analysis. The unfortunate result is sparse knowledge about patterns and trajectories of change, even though some data sets contain suitable data.

Demographers do not have ample skills for detecting and analyzing patterns. We can find help for handling such data. Molecular biologists have devoted great

---

[1] The challenge of studying large numbers of possible patterns at a single time point or over multiple time points (waves) inhibits researchers. They condense the enterprise by reducing disability details or time points. Strategies used to do that are described here. For disability details, (1) disability patterns at a single time point can be summarized into several grades (Anderson et al. 1998). This approach is common in large-scale longitudinal studies, where people are scored in their worst state (institutionalized, any ADL, any IADL, no ADL/IADL) at each wave. (2) Disabilities at each wave can be counted, and changes in patterns of counts are analyzed (Rudberg et al. 1996). (3) Sample means can be generated at each time point, and trajectories of the means studied (Jette et al. 1987; Maddox and Clark, 1992; Verbrugge et al. 1994). (4) Individual trajectories can be reviewed and assigned to qualitative groups such as "steady" or "deteriorate" (Bowling et al. 1994; Charlton, 1989; Fortinsky et al. 1999; Magaziner et al. 1990; also Clipp et al. 1992 for health transitions). (5) Particular trajectories of keen interest can be plucked for study (Ferrucci et al. 1996). The problem of many time points occurs less often because large-scale longitudinal disability studies typically have just a few. But some longitudinal designs now have many waves, e.g., weekly or monthly measurements for a year or more. (1) Wave-to-wave changes can be pooled together, effectively creating a single transition (Mendes de Leon et al. 1999). (2) Individual trajectories can be numerically summarized by standard deviations or means (Verbrugge and Balaban, 1989; Verbrugge et al. 1994) or directly modeled (Beckett et al. 1996). (3) Crafting qualitative patterns (described earlier) also handles the many-waves problem. Three studies maintain full detail of patterns and time points (Dunlop et al. 1997; Verbrugge et al. 2004; Wolinsky et al. 2000) (please inform author of others). Dunlop et al. (1997) show that individuals tend to acquire disabilities in a hierarchical way over time. Verbrugge et al. (2004) find that, of all possible patterns of disability, only a few are common and they are usually hierarchical. Wolinsky et al. (2000) study patterns of functional limitations and how their prevalence changes over waves; several subgroups with specific patterns are traced forward from baseline and backward from last wave.

effort to gene-sequencing methodology. The applicability of gene-sequencing techniques to social science data has been addressed (Abbott, 1995; Dijkstra and Taris, 1995). For data with many-wave measures of functioning, some analog to such techniques will be required to study patterns. Social scientists can learn from gene-sequencing methods and software to tackle the issue of functional trajectories.

Data sources that can inform us about functional trajectories include retrospective studies of last years/months of life, descriptive trajectories of frail older persons, and longitudinal studies with close-in-time re-measurements. The literature is not reviewed fully here; some entrées into it are noted (Gill and Kurland, 2003; Glaser and Strauss, 1968; Guralnik et al. 1991; 1999; Lunney et al. 2003; Verbrugge et al. 1994). Existing multiwave longitudinal studies also have good potential, but their analytic emphasis has been wave-to-wave change rather than full patterns of change.

I end this section by noting there is literature on frailty that does not really fit the topic. First, some articles measure frailty by its consequences. The indicators are physical performance tests (actions such as lifting, reaching, walking), assistance for personal care (ADL) and household management (IADL) tasks, difficulty doing ADL/IADLs due to health, self-rated health, and causes of death. This often happens early in research on a topic, when direct measurements are unavailable or conceptualization is weak. The main problem is if frailty (X) is defined by its consequences, those items can no longer be used as outcomes (Y). This approach greatly limits predictive analyses, and can confuse later researchers. Some of the articles are excellent empirical studies, even if they do not measure frailty directly. Second, because the term is now fashionable, there are articles that claim to study frailty but lack relevant content.

## Frailty in animal models

Frailty's status is markedly different in research on animal models of aging.

Although biology researchers routinely observe animals' late-life impairments and function, the topics are not part of formal data collection and analysis. When asked about their very-long-lived subjects, researchers describe them with brevity. For example: "Aging [of insects] prominently involves the loss of body parts, from wing panels to legs" (Rose et al. 2004). Another example from a workshop discussion: "They [*Drosophila melanogaster*] look about the same, but fly and walk less. ("Do they weigh less?") Yes. ("Do they see less well?") I don't know [pause]. Their parts fall off" (University of Michigan, 2004). Old worms [*C. elegans*] curl up, move slowly and wander, and cannot be stimulated to move (ibid.). Biologists use lay terms such as "decrepit" and "withered" to describe the very old animals. Yet there are sometimes statements about very old "perky" animals (Rose, 1999). Further, current laboratory practices may drop some frail animals from a study population. Subjects that die young, or manage to wander out of the cage/dish environment, are excluded from analysis. For example, worms whose erratic behavior leads them off the plate are ignored in data analyses (University of Michigan, 2004).

Change is occurring in several animal models. A current rodent study includes physiological and functional items, such as bone density, cataract, body weight, hormone and serum levels, and more (P.I.: R.A. Miller, University of Michigan). A current primate study includes measures of wound healing, occurrence and intensity of motion, coarse and fine motor function, short-term memory and executive function, and more (see Ingram et al. 2005). The primate study also includes morbidity and cause of death assessments. Both are long-term omnibus projects, with great forthcoming yield. Aspects of late-life function are entering work on *C. elegans* (Arantes-Oliveira et al. 2003). For medflies (*Ceratitis capitata*), Carey and colleagues are studying individuals' functional trajectories in relation to time of death (Carey and Papadopoulos, 2005). Their descriptive results surpass in quality and detail anything in the human aging literature. The team also studies supine behavior as a frailty indicator (Papadopoulos et al. 2002). A recent analysis of physical performance in old rats shows that their functional abilities decline over time (Carter et al. 2002; see also Ingram, 2000).[2]

The distinction between impairments and functional limitations must be condensed to "function" in biology research. The big issue is whether anything other than death matters in animal models. Why bother with function? I have heard all of the following four arguments against functional assessments in animal research:

1) the notion of function is irrelevant to animals and animal models;
2) function is relevant but unimportant; only mortality is;
3) function is important but too difficult to measure; and
4) function is definitely important, but elaboration of mortality research has more scientific value.

Whether and how to incorporate function into animal models must be debated among biology researchers. Biologists will incorporate function into animal models of aging when they see payoff within their own fields for studying quality as well as quantity of life.

One stated goal of animal models is to obtain knowledge that can inform human aging. Mortality reduction is central to fulfilling that goal, but good late-life function may be important to complete it. From the stance of demography and public health sciences, it appears that contemporary animal models of extended longevity involve high frailty and disability; if so, that reduces their potential relevance for human aging.

It is worth remembering that demography's own history of health research started with a single-minded emphasis on mortality, and the stretch to measurement of physiological and functional aspects of health occurred much later. Mortality is easy to measure. Function takes more time, costs more, and is not feasible until sampling strategies and noninvasive protocols are developed.

---

[2] Desiccation studies of flies could be germane, but their current purpose is to study stress resistance and mortality, not physiologic frailty. The studies typically have severe experimental stimuli, assessments are post-mortem, and analyses are population-level (Graves et al. 1992; Nghiem et al. 2000).

## Crosswalk of demography and biology

Several demography and biology pioneers have discussed genuine links between human research and animal models. Wachter (1997) offers a wide-ranging, compelling discussion of how the two research spheres intertwine. Jazwinski (2002) argues for including measures of frailty and healthy aging in animal models, and for studying individual outcomes as well as population ones. Carey (1997, 2003) informs demographers how current animal models relate to human aging. These crosswalks are huge contributions since scientists on either side seldom pay much attention to each other. The authors above convince us to do otherwise.

There are some fundamental differences between biology and demography that make it difficult to mirror the research designs and practices of one side in the other: First, the timeframes of evolutionary biology and demography differ greatly. Demographic data derive from surveys and clinical evaluations of people living right now (cross-sectional) or for awhile (longitudinal). The questions posed and the answers obtained are tightly circumscribed to current and near-past persons and populations, and future inferences are for near-future only. We are inherently short-sighted compared to evolutionary biology research. Second, biology models of aging focus on population outcomes, such as mortality parameters and trajectories. Demography and public health research on the aging process focus prominently, but not solely, on individual outcomes. To study frailty as described herein, an individual focus is required. It is the only way that the links between frailty, function, and mortality can be measured with certainty. That approach is operationally difficult in many biological studies, especially with numerous, very small subjects. Third, longitudinal data are necessary to study trajectories of frailty and function. Biology has a tremendous advantage since its subjects are caged and always near at hand. Although tagging individuals for identification may be quite a task, follow-ups for function and death assessment are less costly in time and effort than for demographic samples. Fourth, biologists can more readily study the whole life course of subjects than demographers can. Early- and mid-life characteristics can be related to late-life ones more easily in biological studies.

The best inspiration that demography and public health sciences can give to biology will come from richer research on frailty in their own disciplines. First, clarity about conceptual boundaries of frailty should be maintained and reiterated in publications. There is good consensus that frailty's conceptual niche is impairments. Item sets can vary among researchers; in my view, standardization is not needed. Second, the distinguishing features of frailty need to be identified and replicated. They can be signs or symptoms; both fit the concept. The toughest task ahead is to package the features into a syndrome. How are the specific features combined into one or more subsets that define frailty? Third, we need devices to measure functional patterns and trajectories. We can get help from other disciplines with more expertise in pattern recognition. Then, predictive links between frailty and functional patterns/trajectories can be studied.

The next step for animal models is formal inclusion of functional measures in study design, data collection, and analysis. Given the smallness of some animal subjects, and the risks of affecting their health and longevity by obtaining physiological measures, it is likely that behavioral ones will be used first or foremost. Aggregate descriptions of function for age groups and across populations can be produced, and compared with aggregate mortality descriptions. Individual-level relationships of function and mortality can also be studied.

## Conclusion

An ultimate purpose of animal models of aging is obtaining knowledge that informs human aging. Contemporary studies of yeast, *C. elegans, drosophila*, mice, and nonhuman primates focus on identifying genes and dietary/environmental modifications that increase life expectancy. Remarkable increases in population life expectancies have been achieved by particular genetic and "lifestyle" modifications (Jazwinski, 1996, 1998; Magwere et al. 2004; Rose et al. 2004; Wachter and Finch, 1997). These findings have delighted biologists, and implications for the human model of aging are sometimes advanced.

The public health goal for human populations is long lives in tandem with good function and physiological resilience. When asked, biologists say that very-long-lived flies, worms, and others are inactive, seldom move voluntarily, or wander aimlessly when they do move. Flies' wings atrophy and fall off. These features are considered unimportant and are rarely formally recorded as data. Thus, contemporary animal models of extended longevity seem to include high disability and frailty. We will not know for sure if that is true, or not true, until function becomes a key aspect of biological studies.

Within demography, novel but empirically feasible measures of frailty and functional trajectories are needed in studies of older persons. Crosswalks between demography and biology can be strengthened by each side reading the other's literature and looking for new ideas or hypotheses. These steps may inspire new designs and data collection in biology that focus on both frailty and mortality outcomes. Are there models of longevous agile worms and long-lived flies with wings waiting to be discovered? Probably so, and they will inform human aging in profound ways.

## References

Abbott A (1995) A comment on 'Measuring the agreement between sequences'. Sociolog Meth Res 24: 232– 243

Anderson RT, James M, Miller ME, Worley AS, Longino CF (1998) The timing of change: patterns in transitions in functional status among elderly persons. J GerontolSoc Sci 53B: S17– S27

Arantes-Oliveira N, Berman JR, Kenyon C (2003) Healthy animals with extreme longevity. Science 302: 611

Bales CW, Ritchie CS (2002) Sarcopenia, weight loss, and nutritional frailty in the elderly. Ann Rev Nutr 22: 309– 323

Baltes PB, Smith J (2003) New frontiers in the future of aging: from successful aging of the young old to the dilemmas of the fourth age. Gerontology 49: 123– 135

Barron JS, Duffey PL, Byrd LJ, Campbell R, Ferrucci L (2004) Informed consent for research participation in frail older persons. Aging – Clin Exp Res 16:79– 85

Beckett LA, Brock DB, Lemke JH, Mendes de Leon CF, Guralnik JM, Fillenbaum GG, Branch LG, Wetle TT, Evans DA (1996) Analysis of change in self-reported physical function among older persons in four population studies. Am J Epidemiol 143: 766– 778

Bennett AK (2004) Older age underwriting: frisky vs frail. J Insurance Med 36: 74– 83

Binder EF, Schechtman KB, Ehsani AA, Steger-May K, Brown M, Sinacore DR, Yarasheski KE, Holloszy JO (2002) Effects of exercise training on frailty in community-dwelling older adults: results of a randomized, controlled trial. J Am Geriat Soc 50: 1921– 1928

Black SA, Rush RD (2002) Cognitive and functional decline in adults aged 75 and older. J Am Geriat Soc 50: 1978– 1986

Bortz WM 2d (1993) The physics of frailty. J Am Geriat Soc 41: 1004– 1008

Bowling S, Farquhar M, Grundy E (1994) Associations with changes in level of functional ability. Results from a follow-up survey at two and a half years of people ages 85 years and over at baseline interview. Ageing Soc 14: 53– 73

Carey JR (1997) What demographers can learn from fruit fly actuarial models and biology. Demography 34: 17–30

Carey JR (2003). Longevity. The biology and demography of life span. Princeton, New Jersey: Princeton University Press

Carey JR, Papadopoulos N (2005) The Medfly as a frailty model: implications for biodemographic research. In: Carey J, Robine JM, Michel JP, Christen Y, eds: Longevity and frailty. Heidelberg.Springer Verlag, pp.

Carter CS, Sonntag WE, Onder G, Pahor M (2002) Physical performance and longevity in aged rats. J Gerontol – Biol Sci 57A: B193–B197

Charlton JRH (1989). Measuring disability in a longitudinal survey. In: Patrick DL, Peach H (eds) Disablement in the community. Oxford: Oxford University Press, pp. 62–80

Chin A, Paw MJ, de Groot LC, van Gend SV, Schoterman MH, Schouten EG, Schroll M, van Staveren WA (2003) Inactivity and weight loss; effective criteria to identify frailty. J Nutr Health Aging 7: 55–60

Clipp EC, Pavalko EK, Elder GH Jr (1992) Trajectories of health: in concept and empirical pattern. Behav Health Aging 2: 159–179

Cohen HJ (2000) In search of the underlying mechanisms of frailty. J Gerontol – Med Sci 55A(12): M706–M708

Covinsky KE, Eng C, Lui LY, Sands LP, Yaffe K (2003) The last 2 years of life: functional trajectories of frail older people. J Am Geriat Soc 51: 492–498

Dijkstra W, Taris T (1995) Measuring the agreement between sequences. Sociolog Meth Res 24: 214–231

Dunlop DD, Hughes SL, Manheim LM (1997) Disability in activities of daily living: patterns of change and a hierarchy of disability. Am J Publ Health 87: 378–383

Felten BS, Hall JM (2001) Conceptualizing resilience in women older than 85: overcoming adversity from illness or loss. J Gerontol Nurs 27: 46–53

Ferrucci L, Ble A, Bandinelli S, Windham G, Simonsick EM (2005) Inflammation: the fire of frailty. In: Carey J, Robine JM, Michel JP, Christen Y, eds: Longevity and frailty. Heidelberg: Springer Verlag, pp. 91–98

Ferrucci L, Guralnik JM, Simonsick E, Salive ME, Corti C, Langlois J (1996) Progressive versus catastrophic disability: a longitudinal view of the disablement process. J Gerontol – Med Sci 51A: M123–M130

Ferrucci L, Cavazzini C, Corsi A, Bartali B, Russo CR, Lauretani F, Ferrucci L, Cavazzini C, Corsi AM, Bartali B, Russo CR, Lauretani F, Bandinelli S, Bandinelli S, Guralnik JM (2002) Biomarkers of frailty in older persons. J Endocrinol Invest 25 (10 Suppl): 10–15

Ferrucci L, Guralnik JM, Cavazzini C, Bandinelli S, Laurentani F, Bartali B, Repetto L, Longo DL (2003) The frailty syndrome: a critical issue in geriatric oncology. Crit Rev Oncol – Hematol 46: 127–137

Ferrucci L, Guralnik JM, Studenski S, Fried LP, Cutler GB Jr, Walston JD (Interventions on Frailty Working Group) (2004) Designing randomized, controlled trials aimed at preventing or delaying functional decline and disability in frail, older persons: a consensus report. J Am Geriat Soc 52(4): 625–634

Fortinsky RH, Covinsky KE, Palmer RM, Landefeld CS (1999). Effects of functional status changes before and during hospitalization on nursing home admission of older adults. JGerontol – Med Sci, 54A, M521–M526

Fried LP, Walston J (1999) Frailty and failure to thrive. In: Hazzard WR, Blass JP, Ettinger WH, Halter JB, Ouslander JG (eds) Principles of geriatric medicine and gerontology. Fourth Edition. New York: McGraw Hill, pp. 1387–1402

Fried LP, Tangen CM, Walston J, Newman AB, Hirsch C, Gottdiener J, Seeman T, Tracy R, Kop WJ, Burke G, McBurnie MA (Cardiovascular Health Study Collaborative Research Group) (2001) Frailty in older adults: evidence for a phenotype. J Gerontol – Med Sci 56A: M145–M156

Fried LP, Ferrucci L, Darer J, Williamson JD, Anderson G (2004) Untangling the concepts of disability, frailty, and comorbidity: implications for improved targeting and care. J Gerontol – Med Sci 59A(3): 255–263

Gessert CE, Elliott BA, Haller IV (2002) Dying of old age: an examination of death certificates of Minnesota centenarians. J Am Geriat Soc 50: 1561–1565

Gill TM, Kurland B (2003) The burden and patterns of disability in activities of daily living among community-living older persons. J Gerontol – Med Sciences 58A: 70–75

Glaser B, Strauss AL (1968) Time for dying. Chicago, Illinois: Aldine Publishing Co.

Graves JL, Toolson EC, Jeong C, Vu LN, Rose MR (1992) Desiccation, flight, glycogen, and postponed senescence in *drosophila melanogaster*. Physiol Zoology 65: 268–286

Guralnik JM, LaCroix AZ, Branch LG, Kasl SV, Wallace RB (1991) Mortality and disability in older persons in the years prior to death. Am J Publ Health 81: 443–447

Guralnik JM, Ferrucci L, Penninx BW, Kasper JD, Leveille SG, Bandeen-Roche K, Fried LP (1999) New and worsening conditions and change in physical and cognitive performance during weekly evaluations over 6 months: the Women's Health and Aging Study. J Gerontol – Med Sci 54A:M410–422

Hadley EC, Ory MG, Suzman R, Weindruch R, Fried L (eds) (1993) Symposium on physical frailty. A treatable cause of dependence in old age. J Gerontol 48 (Special issue)

Hamerman D (1999) Toward an understanding of frailty. Ann Intern Med 130: 945–950

Hardy SE, Gill TM (2004) Recovery from disability among community-dwelling older persons. JAMA 291: 1596–1602

Hogan DB, MacKnight C, Bergman H (Steering Committee, Canadian Initiative on Frailty and Aging) (2003) Models, definitions, and criteria of frailty. Aging – ClinExpResearch 15(3 Suppl): 1–29

Imuta H, Yasumura S, Abe H, Fukao A (2001) The prevalence and psychosocial characteristics of the frail elderly in Japan: a community-based study. Aging – Clin Exp Res 13: 443–453

Ingram DK (2000) Age-related decline in physical activity: generalization to nonhumans. Med Sci Sports Exercise 32: 1623–1629

Ingram DK, de Cabo R, Anson N, Ottinger MA, Lane MA, Roth GS, Mattison JA (2005) Calorie restriction in nonhuman primates: impact on aging, disease, and frailty. In: Carey J, Robine J-M, Michel J-M, Christen Y, eds : Longevity and frailty. Heidelberg: Springer Verlag, pp. 39–56

Interagency Committee on Disability Research (2004) Workshop on best practices for surveying people with disabilities. Washington, D.C., Interagency Subcommittee on Disability Statistics, National Institute on Disability and Rehabilitation Research

Jazwinski SM (1996) Longevity, genes, and aging. Science 273: 54–59

Jazwinski SM (1998) Genetics of longevity. Exp Gerontol 33: 773–783

Jazwinski SM (2002) Biological aging research today: potential, peeves, and problems. Exp Gerontol 37: 1141–1146

Jette AM, Harris BA, Cleary PD, Campion EW (1987) Functional recovery after hip fracture. Arch Phys Med Rehab 68: 735–740

Kinney JM (2004) Nutritional frailty, sarcopenia and falls in the elderly. Curr Opin Clin Nutrit Metab Care 7: 15–20

Lamberts SWJ, van den Beld AW, van der Lely AJ (1997) The endocrinology of aging. Science 278: 419–424

Lipsitz LA (2002) Dynamics of stability: the physiologic basis of functional health and frailty. J Gerontol – Biol Sci 57A: B115–B125

Lipsitz LA (2004) Physiological complexity, aging, and the path to frailty. Sci Aging Knowl Environ 2004(16, 21 Apr): 16

Lunney JR, Lynn J, Hogan C (2002) Profiles of older Medicare decedents. J Am Geriat Soc 50: 1108–1112

Lunney JR, Lynn J, Foley DJ, Lipson S, Guralnik JM (2003) Patterns of functional decline at the end of life. JAMA 289: 2387–2392

Maddox GL, Clark DO (1992). Trajectories of functional impairment in later life. J Health Soc Behav 33: 114–125

Magaziner J, Simonsick EM, Kashner TM, Hebel JR, Kenzora JE (1990) Predictors of functional recovery one year following hospital discharge for hip fracture: a prospective study. J Gerontol – Med Sci 45: M101–M107

Magwere T, Chapman T, Partridge L (2004) Sex differences in the effect of dietary restriction of life span and mortality rates in female and male drosophila melanogaster. J Gerontol – Biol Sci 59A: B3–B9

Manton KG (1986) Cause specific mortality patterns among the oldest-old: multiple cause of death trends 1968 to 1980. J Gerontol 41: 282–289

Marcell TJ (2003) Sarcopenia: causes, consequences, and prevention. J Gerontol – Medical Sci 58A: M911–M916

Markle-Reid M, Browne G (2003) Conceptualizations of frailty in relation to older adults. J Adv Nurs 44: 58–68

Matthews M, Lucas A, Boland R, Hirth V, Odenheimer G, Wieland D, William H, Elezer GP (2004) Use of a questionnaire to screen for frailty in the elderly: an exploratory study. Aging – ClinExp Res 16: 34–40

Mehdizadeh SA (2002) Health and long-term care use trajectories of older disabled women. The Gerontologist 42: 304–313

Mendes de Leon DF, Glass TA, Beckett LA, Seeman TE, Evans DA, Berkman LF (1999). Social networks and disability transitions across eight intervals of yearly data in the New Haven EPESE. J Gerontol – Soc Sci 54B: S162–S172

Mitnitski AB, Mogilner AJ, Rockwood K (2001) Accumulation of deficits as a proxy measure of aging. Sci World J 1: 323–336

Mitnitski AB, Mogilner AJ, MacKnight C, Rockwood K (2002) The mortality rate as a function of accumulated deficits in a frailty index. Mech Ageing Devel 123: 1457–1460

Mitnitski AB, Song X, Rockwood K (2004) The estimation of relative fitness and frailty in community-dwelling older adults using self-report data. J Gerontol – MedSci 59A: M627–632

Morley JE (2001) Anorexia, sarcopenia, and aging. Nutrition 17: 660–663

Morley JE, Baumgartner RN, Roubenoff R, Mayer J, Nair KS (2001) Sarcopenia. J Lab Clin Med 137: 231–243

Morley JE, Perry HM 3d, Miller DK (2002) Something about frailty. J Gerontol – Med Sci 57A: M698–M704

Muhlberg W, Sieber C (2004) Sarcopenia and frailty in geriatric patients: implications for training and prevention. Zeitschrift Gerontol Geriatrie 37:2–8

National Institute on Aging (2003) Frailty in old age: pathophysiology and interventions. Program announcement PAS-03-122. Bethesda, MD, National Institutes of Health

National Institutes of Health (1991) Physical frailty: a reducible barrier to independence for older Americans. Report to the U.S. Senate Committee on Appropriations. NIH Publ. No. 91-397. Bethesda, MD

Nghiem D, Gibbs AG, Rose MR, Bradley TJ (2000) Postponed aging and desiccation resistance in *drosophila melanogaster*. Exp Gerontol 35: 957–969

Papadopoulos NT, Carey JR, Katsoyannos BI, Kouloussis NA, Muller HG, Liu X (2002) Supine behavior predicts the time to death in male Mediterranean fruitflies (*Ceratitis capitata*). Proc Royal Soc London: Biol Sci 269: 1633–1637

Raphael D, Cava M, Brown I, Renwick R, Heathcote K, Weir N, Wright K, Kirwan L (1995) Frailty: a public health perspective. Can J Publ Health 86: 224–227

Robine JM, Michel JP (2004) Looking forward to a general theory on population aging. JGerontol – Med Sci59A: M590–M597

Rockwood K, Hogan DB, MacKnight C (2000) Conceptualisation and measurement of frailty in elderly people. Drugs Aging 17: 295–302

Rose MR (1999) Can human aging be postponed? Sci Am 281:106–111.

Rose MR, Passananti HB, Matos M (2004) Introduction: why Methuselah flies? In: Rose MR, Passananti HB, Matos M (eds) Methuselah flies. A case study in the evolution of aging. World Scientific Publishing Co., Singapore, pp ix–xiv

Roubenoff R (1999) The pathophysiology of wasting in the elderly. J Nutrit 129(1S Suppl): 256S–259S

Roubenoff R (2000) Sarcopenia: a major modifiable cause of frailty in the elderly. J NutritHealth Aging 4: 140–142

Rudberg MA, Parzen MI, Leonard LA, Cassel CK (1996). Functional limitation pathways and transitions in community-dwelling older persons. The Gerontologist 36: 430–440

Schulz R, Williamson GM (1993) Psychosocial and behavioral dimensions of physical frailty. J Gerontol 48 (Special Issue, Sept): 39–43

Shlipak MG, Stehman-Breen C, Fried LF, Song X, Siscovick D, Fried LP, Psaty BM, Newman AB (2004) The presence of frailty in elderly persons with chronic renal insufficiency. Am J Kidney Dis 43: 861–867

Strawbridge WJ, Shema SJ, Balfour JL, Higby HR, Kaplan GA (1998) Antecedents of frailty over three decades in an older cohort. J Gerontol – Soc Sci 53B:S9–S16

Syddall H, Cooper C, Martin F, Briggs R, Aihie Sayer A (2003) Is grip strength a useful single marker of frailty? Age Ageing 32: 650–656

University of Michigan, Institute of Gerontology (2004) Models systems in the study of aging. Nathan Shock Center 2004 Workshop, 24–25 May. Ann Arbor, Michigan

Vanitallie TB (2003) Frailty in the elderly: contributions of sarcopenia and visceral protein depletion. MetabClin Exp 52 (10 Suppl 2): 22–26

Verbrugge LM, Balaban DJ (1989) Patterns of change in disability and well-being. Med Care 27(3, Supplement): S128–S147

Verbrugge LM, Jette AM (1994) The disablement process. Soc Sci Med 38: 1–14

Verbrugge LM, Reoma JM, Gruber-Baldini AL (1994) Short-term dynamics of disability and well-being. J Health Soc Behav 35: 97–117

Verbrugge LM, Yang L, Juarez L (2004) Severity, timing, and structure of disability. Soc Prevent Med 49: 110–121

Wachter KW (1997) Between Zeus and the salmon: introduction. In: Wachter KE, Finch CE (eds) Between Zeus and the salmon. The biodemography of longevity. National Academy Press, Washington, D.C., pp 1–16

Wachter KE, Finch CE (eds) Between Zeus and the salmon. The biodemography of longevity. National Academy Press, Washington, D.C.

Walston J (2004) Frailty -- the search for underlying causes. Sci Aging Knowl Environ2004 (28 January): 4

Walston J (2005) Biological markers and molecular biology of frailty. In: Carey J, Robine J-M, Michel J-P, Christen Y, eds : Longevity and frailty. Heidelberg: Springer Verlag, pp. 83–90

Walston J, Fried LP (1999) Frailty and the older man. Med Clin North Am 83(5): 1173–1194

Walston J, McBurnie MA, Newman A, Tracy RP, Kop WJ, Hirsch CH, Gottdiener J, Fried LP (Cardiovascular Health Study) (2002) Frailty and activation of the inflammation and coagulation systems with and without clinical comorbidities: results from the Cardiovascular Health Study. Arch Intern Med 162: 2333–2341

Wells JL, Seabrook JA, Stolee P, Borrie MJ, Knoefel F (2003) State of the art in geriatric rehabilitation. Part I: review of frailty and comprehensive geriatric assessment. Arch Phys Med Rehab 84: 890–897

Winograd CH, Gerety MB, Chung M, Goldstein MK, Dominguez F Jr, Vallone R (1991) Screening for frailty: criteria and predictors of outcomes. J Am Geriat Soc 39: 778–784

Wolinsky FD, Armbrecht ES, Wyrwich KW (2000) Rethinking functional limitation pathways. The Gerontologist 40: 137–146

# Biological Markers and the Molecular Biology of Frailty

*Jeremy D. Walston*[1]

Frailty has been difficult to characterize because of its biologic complexity and because it frequently overlaps with medical illness and disability. We recently validated a frailty screening exam based on muscle weakness, slow walking speed, fatigue, weight loss, and low activity levels. Those who were deemed frail by these criteria were more likely to be hospitalized, develop disability, and die earlier than those who were not frail. Further cross-sectional studies of frail older adults (deemed frail by these validated criteria) have demonstrated strong relationships between frailty and alterations in specific biological markers that represent multiple physiologic systems. These include increased markers of inflammation, such as IL-6, CRP, total white blood cells, and monocytes, as well as increased acute phase reactants and markers of the clotting process, including fibrinogen, Factor VIII, and D-dimers, in frail compared to non-frail older adults. Several other biomarkers of metabolism are also altered in frailty, with evidence for decreased glucose tolerance, lower levels of IGF-1, and lower levels of DHEA-S all associated with frailty. Some interactions between endocrine and inflammatory systems have been studied, with evidence suggesting that inflammation may be in part influencing changes in the endocrine systems. These early cross-sectional studies have helped to better characterize the multiple physiologic and molecular systems that may be involved in the development of frailty. They also highlight the potential importance of NfκB-related inflammatory system activation. Future studies focused on the interactions between physiological systems, the development of tissue-specific biomarkers to help determine the source of inflammatory biomarkers (i.e., fat, endothelial cells, immune system, fibroblasts), the development of cumulative measures that better gauge risk of frailty and poor outcomes, and the investigation of molecular triggering mechanisms for inflammation may help lead to the discovery of etiologies and the development of prevention and treatment for frailty.

[1] Associate Professor of Medicine, Division of Geriatric Medicine and Gerontology, Johns Hopkins University School of Medicine, JHAAC Rm. 5A.24, 5505 Bayview Circle, Baltimore, MD 21224, 410-550-1003, e-mail: jwaltson@jhmi.edu

Carey et al.
Longevity and Frailty

## Conceptualization of Frailty

Frailty in humans is an intuitive concept that has long helped family members, caregivers, and physicians describe a subset of older adults who appear to be at greatest risk of falling, developing medical complications, losing independence, and dying. This concept has been difficult to characterize for research purposes because of the complexity of the underlying physiology that drives frailty, and because of the frequent overlap between disease states (co-morbidity), disability, and frailty. Many previous definitions of human frailty have in fact included specific diseases and disabilities in the definition. Frailty is almost certainly related to clinical and subclinical diseases that can be confounders, modifiers, or etiologic and must be accounted for in any development of frailty studies. To begin to differentiate the biology that underlies frailty from the biology of specific disease states, we developed a conceptual model of frailty that includes a central cycle of decline in skeletal muscle (sarcopenia), energy expenditure, and nutrition that then impacts on function via declines in strength, power and ambulatory ability, which in turn feeds back into the central cycle of decline (Fig. 1). It is apparent that this cycle can be affected by external triggers, such as injuries, medical

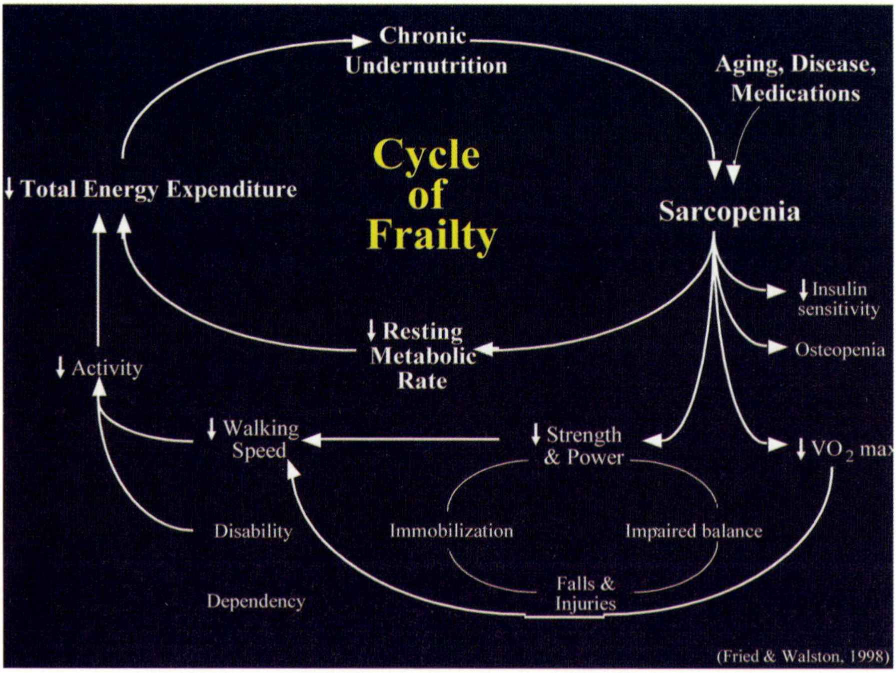


**Fig. 1.** Hypothetical cycle of frailty that demonstrates a central cycle of physiologic and environmental change that directly influences functional decline and the development of disability (adapted from Principles of Geriatric Medicine and Gerontology, Chapter 109, 1998).

illnesses, medications, and psychosocial stressors, and perhaps by aging-related biologic decline as well.

## Development of a Frailty Phenotype

To better understand the biology of frailty, it was necessary to develop, put into operation, and validate a frailty screening exam. Based on clinical findings of frail older adults, a screening exam was developed and tested in the Cardiovascular Health Study population. All those with Parkinson's disease, severe cognitive deficits, depression, and CVA with hemiparesis were excluded from the analysis (Fried et al. 2001). The presence of three or more of five criteria for frailty, including weight loss, weakness, exhaustions, slow walking speed, and low levels of physical activity, significantly predicted the onset of falls (HR 1.26, CI 1.00-1.68), mobility declines (HR 1.50; CI 1.23-1.82), worsening ADL disability (HR 1.98, 1.54-2.55), and death (HR 2.24; CI 1.51-3.33) over a period of three years, even after adjustment for age, race, educational background, and several disease and health measurements (Fried et al. 2001). Importantly, those individuals who met one or two of the frailty criteria were also at increased risk for developing frailty and for poor outcomes, further establishing the validity of this screening exam (Fried et al. 2001). These validated criteria may serve as an important starting point from which to test other, more phenotypic and/or biologic frailty screening criteria, including those that include measures of cognitive impairment. In addition, these criteria have proven to be an outstanding starting point in the characterization of the multiple physiologic and biologic systems thought to be altered in frailty.

## Specific biomarkers and biology of frailty

Building on literature and evidence developed by investigators who have studied wasting diseases and multisystemic decline, we have developed hypothetical pathways that are most likely operant in frailty, including the activation of inflammation, altered neuroendocrine systems, and declines in skeletal muscle that all

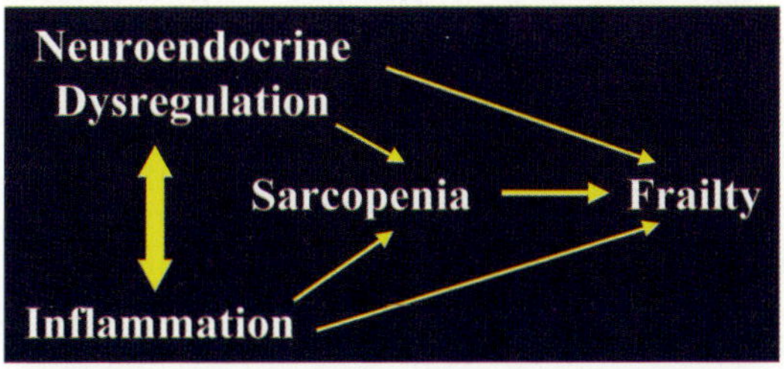


Fig. 2. Physiologic systems (neuroendocrine and inflammatory) hypothesized to influence both skeletal muscle declines (sarcopenia) and ultimately frailty.

contribute to the development of frailty (Buchner and Wagner 1992; Roubenoff 1997). Figure 2 shows a conceptual model of the physiologic changes and interactions that we hypothesize underlie frailty.

## Inflammation and Frailty

Using the frailty phenotype developed in the Cardiovascular Health Study population, we tested the hypothesis that frailty correlates with serum measurements that reflect the activation of inflammatory pathways. Indeed, we have identified several important correlates of inflammation in this population, including significantly increased C-reactive protein, fibrinogen, and Factor VIII (Walston et al. 2002). We found that these measurements were also higher in the intermediate frail population and that the statistical differences remained unchanged when those with diabetes and cardiovascular disease were excluded from the analyses. In a related analyses, we also identified mean increased fasting and two-hour glucose and insulin (after oral glucose tolerance test) values that were significantly higher in frail compared to non-frail individuals, further supporting metabolic change potentially related to inflammation (Walston et al. 2002). Other findings from this study included significantly higher levels of d-dimer along with increased fibrinogen and Factor VIII in frail compared to non-frail adults in a subset of this population, suggesting the activation of clotting pathways in frailty (Walston et al. 2002).

These findings of increased inflammation in frailty have been further validated by Leng et al. (2002) in a smaller study of frail compared to non-frail older adults. After age and disease status adjustment, the frail, older adults had a significantly higher level of the inflammatory cytokine IL-6 (4.4 + 2.9 vs. 2.8 + 1.6 pg/ul , $p = 0.03$). In addition, a relationship was identified between lower levels of hemoglobin and frailty, as well as an inverse relationship between increased IL-6 and lower hemoglobin in the frail but not the non-frail in this population (Leng et al. 2002). IL-6 is an important inflammatory cytokine that acts as a transcription factor; when chronically elevated, it has negative clinical impacts on bone, muscle, and stem cells (Ershler and Keller 2000). In addition, increased levels of serum IL-6 have previously been associated with the development of disability and mortality in older adults (Ferrucci et al. 1999; Harris et al. 1999). Finally, in an ex vivo study that utilized the same screening exam to identify frail and control subjects, the reaction of mononuclear blood cells to lipopolysaccharide (LPS) was studied. In this study, mononuclear cells extracted from frail older adults secreted significantly more IL-6 after (LPS) stimulation, which reached statistical significance at 48 hours (Fig. 3; Leng et al. 2004). This pilot study finding supports the hypothesis that altered immune system function characterized by increased reactivity to immunologic stressors is operant in frailty and provides further rationale for the study of immune system differences between frail and non-frail older adults.

Although the association studies on frailty have been cross-sectional to date, they have helped to establish inflammation as a characteristic of frailty and have helped to demonstrate that specific immune system cells may play an important role in this inflammatory change. In addition, these data serve as preliminary evi-

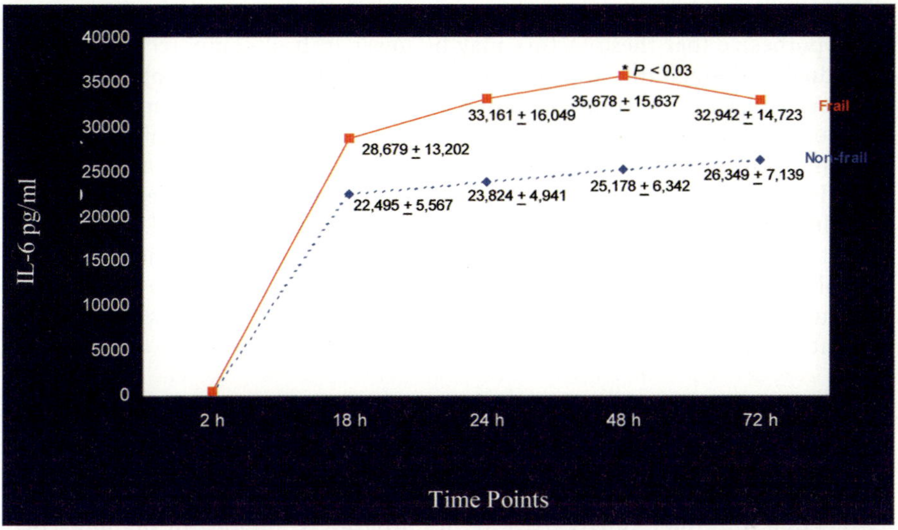


**Fig. 3.** Mean IL-6 levels as measured from LPS-stimulated immune system mononuclear cells from frail (red line) subjects (n=11) and non-frail (blue line) age- and gender-matched control subjects (n=11). The difference in IL-6 levels reached statistical significance at 48 hours after LPS stimulation ($p < 0.03$).

dence that supports further exploration of specific components of inflammatory pathways, immune system cells, and inflammation triggers that may be important in the development of frailty.

## Endocrine Biomarkers of Frailty

As illustrated in Figure 2, we previously hypothesized that hormones related to skeletal muscle mass maintenance might be decreased in frail, older adults. We tested this hypothesis in a smaller cohort of frail and non-frail older adults using baseline blood and serum data. Cappola et al. (2001) previously demonstrated an association between lower levels of muscle strength and of insulin-like growth factor -1 (IGF-1) in older, disabled women. IGF-1 is the first messenger molecule directly related to growth hormone secretion (Thompson et al. 1995). Dehydroepiandrosterone-Sulfate (DHEA-S) is an adrenal androgen and appears to play an important role in the protection of skeletal muscle and other tissues from inflammatory changes via blocking NfkB-induced inflammation pathways (Allolio and Arlt 2002; Aragno et al. 2002). We hypothesized that these hormones would be lower in frail compared to non-frail subjects. Age-adjusted analyses from 18 frail and 33 non-frail subjects found significantly lower serum levels of IGF-1 (88+49 vs. 122 + 47, p = 0.023) and DHEA-S (0.30 + 0.21 vs. 0.53+ 0.25, p = 0.016). Other potential bioactive endocrine factors that are known to impact skeletal muscle, change with age, and potentially interact with inflammatory mediators such as IL-

6 include testosterone and estrogen (Ershler and Keller 2000; Morley et al. 1997). We hypothesize that these factors may be lower in frail compared to non-frail individuals, although this idea remains to be tested using a frailty phenotype. Finally, cortisol, a critical component of the hypothalamic-pituitary-adrenal (HPA) axis, becomes increasingly dysregulated, negatively impacts skeletal muscle, and likely increases in older adults (Seeman and Robbins 1994). This induced stress steroid hormone is also an important candidate for a bioactive molecular marker of frailty in older adults. The pilot study results reported above and the potential candidate hormones will need to be further tested in cross-sectional and longitudinal populations with more individuals and with inflammatory measures to begin to better understand individual and interactive contributions to the development of frailty.

## Towards a better understanding of the molecular biology of frailty

As research into the biomarkers of frailty progresses, interest in the molecular basis of these physiologic changes is increasing. It is likely that the physiologic changes observed in the frail cohort are not frailty-specific: it is likely that both

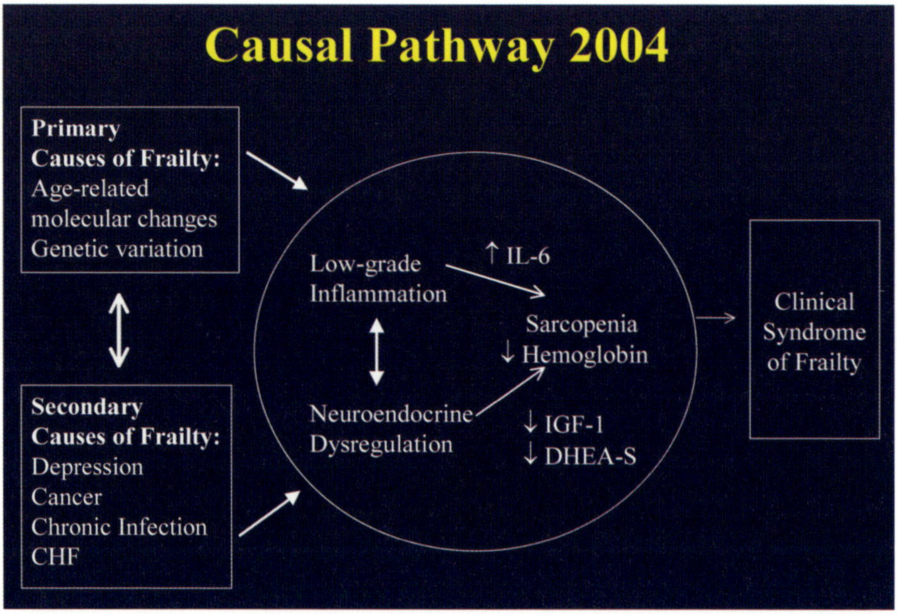


**Fig. 4.** Hypothetical causal pathway towards frailty, with central circle representing physiologic pathways and specific biomarkers that are related to frailty. The boxes on the left demonstrate primary or age-related alterations that may have an impact on frailty, and secondary, or disease-related triggers that likely affect the same physiology and, ultimately, frailty (adapted from Palliative Care Text, 2003)

chronic disease states and genetic polymorphisms, along with age-related molecular changes, can contribute to this altered physiologic state. Figure 4 represents a hypothetical causal pathway, with possible triggering mechanisms represented by the boxes entitled primary (age-induced) and secondary (disease-induced) frailty. Possible candidates that might trigger frailty and warrant further study include mitochondrial change, cumulative oxidative damage, and related DNA damage (Souza-Pinto and Bohr 2002). In addition, telomere loss and the increasing burden of senescent cells can induce abnormal protein production and increase secretion of inflammatory cytokines IL-6 and IL-1, warranting further exploration (Campisi 2003; Kim et al. 2002). Finally, genetic polymorphisms in hundreds of genes, including those that have an impact on oxidative damage protection, cell senescence, inflammation, specific endocrine pathways, and skeletal muscle mass maintenance, may all affect the development of frailty late in life and could potentially be important in the identification of critical molecular pathways that contribute to frailty.

## Next steps in frailty research

As the understanding of the physiology and molecular biology of frailty increases in the coming years, it will be of critical importance to improve the measurement of frailty and its predictors, including cognitive measures, physiologic predictors, and outcomes. In addition, as the understanding of the biological systems involved in vulnerability progresses, studies that develop provocative tests and those that identify critical risk periods and triggering mechanisms will be necessary. Given that so many interactive physiologic and molecular systems play a role in the development and propagation of frailty, improved biostatistical models and high-quality data from longitudinal studies will need to be accessed. In addition, the development of cellular and animal models that target late life changes will help identify potentially important molecular and physiologic pathways in humans. Further development and testing of hypothetical connections between important basic aging changes, such as oxidative stress, cell senescence, and telomere shortening, and physiologic changes, such as increased inflammation and endocrine system decline, will greatly facilitate a translational research agenda and lead to improved preventive and intervention strategies in older adults (Walston 2004).

## References

Allolio B, Arlt W (2002) DHEA treatment: myth or reality? Trends Endocrinol Metab 13(7):288-294.

Aragno M, Mastrocola R, Brignardello E, Catalano M, Robino G, Manti R, Parola M, Danni O, Boccuzzi G (2002) Dehydroepiandrosterone modulates nuclear factor-kappaB activation in hippocampus of diabetic rats. Endocrinology 143:3250-3258.

Buchner DM, Wagner EH (1992) Preventing frail health. Clin Geriatr Med 1992; 8(1):1-17.

Campisi J (2003) Cellular senescence and apoptosis: how cellular responses might influence aging phenotypes. Exp Gerontol 38:5-11.

Cappola AR, Bandeen-Roche K, Wand GS, Volpato S, Fried LP (2001) Association of IGF-I levels with muscle strength and mobility in older women. J Clin Endocrinol Metab 86(9):4139-4146. Ershler WB, Keller ET (2000) Age-associated increased interleukin-6 gene expression, late-life diseases, and frailty. Annu Rev Med 51:245-270.

Ferrucci L, Harris TB, Guralnik JM, Tracy RP, Corti MC, Cohen HJ, Penninx B, Pahor M, Wallace R, Havlik RJ (1999) Serum IL-6 level and the development of disability in older persons. J Am Geriatr Soc 47:639-646.

Fried LP, Tangen C, Walston J, Newman A, Hirsch CH, Gottdiener JS, Seeman T, Tracy R, Kop WJ, Burke G, McBurnie MA, Cardiovascular Health Study Collaborative Research Group (2001) Frailty in older adults: evidence for a phenotype. J Gerontol 56A: M146-156

Harris TB, Ferrucci L, Tracy RP, Corti MC, Wacholder S, Ettinger WH, Jr. Heimovitz H, Cohen HJ, Wallace R (1999) Associations of elevated interleukin-6 and C-reactive protein levels with mortality in the elderly. Am J Med 106:506-512.

Kim Sh SH, Kaminker P, Campisi J (2002) Telomeres, aging and cancer: in search of a happy ending. Oncogene 21:503-511.

Leng S, Chaves P, Koenig K, Walston J (2002) Serum interleukin-6 and hemoglobin as physiological correlates in the geriatric syndrome of frailty: a pilot study. J Am Geriatr Soc 50:1268-1271.

Leng S, Huanle Y, Walston J (2004) Decreased cell proliferation and altered cytokine production in frail older adults. Aging Clin Exp Res 16:249-252.

Morley JE, Kaiser FE, Perry HM, III, Patrick P, Morley PM, Stauber PM, Vellas B, Baumgartner RN, Garry PJ (1997) Longitudinal changes in testosterone, luteinizing hormone, and follicle-stimulating hormone in healthy older men. Metabolism 46:410-413.

Roubenoff R (1997) Inflammatory and hormonal mediators of cachexia. J Nutr 127(5 Suppl):1014S-1016S.

Seeman TE, Robbins RJ (1994) Aging and hypothalamic-pituitary-adrenal response to challenge in humans. Endocr Rev 15:233-260.

Souza-Pinto NC, Bohr VA (2002) The mitochondrial theory of aging: involvement of mitochondrial DNA damage and repair. Int Rev Neurobiol 53:519-534.

Thompson JL, Butterfield GE, Marcus R, Hintz RL, Van Loan M, Ghiron L, Hoffman AR (1995) The effects of recombinant human insulin-like growth factor-I and growth hormone on body composition in elderly women. J Clin Endocrinol Metab 80:1845-1852.

Walston J (2004) Frailty--the search for underlying causes. Sci Aging Knowledge Environ 2004(4):e4.

Walston J, McBurnie MA, Newman A, Tracy R, Kop WJ, Hirsch CH, Gottdiener J, Fried LP, Cardiovascular Health Study (2002) Frailty and activation of the inflammation and coagulation systems with and without clinical morbidities: Results from the Cardiovascular Health Study. Arch Intern Med 162:2333-2341.

# Inflammation: the fire of frailty?

*Luigi Ferrucci*[1], *Alessandro Ble*[1], *Stefania Bandinelli*[2], *B Gwen Windham*[1], *Eleanor M Simonsick*[1]

## Aging as progressive biological instability

Aging is associated with biological instability in virtually all living organisms, including humans. This biological instability reduces the capacity for maintaining homeostasis and, thus, for recovery from the destabilizing effects of environmental stressors, which over time result in inevitable multi-system failure and death. Observational studies in representative populations have shown that, relative to younger persons, older persons have an increased risk of developing physical limitations, cognitive impairment, and multiple diseases (Fried et al. 2004; Di Carlo et al. 2000). Moreover, it has been demonstrated that mortality rises exponentially with chronological age (Vaupel et al. 1998). These observations are consistent with a model of aging based on progressive development of biological instability. At present, the molecular mechanisms that underlie this biological instability and its relationship with chronological aging have not been extensively explored. Additionally, although a wealth of data exists on the aging process, both at the cellular and molecular levels and at the physiological and behavioral levels, these two highly interconnected aspects of the aging process have rarely been studied simultaneously. Only recently epidemiological and clinical studies on aging have explored the relationship between biomarkers of inflammation and oxidative stress, two highly prevalent and important pathologic conditions frequently associated with increased rates of decline in physical and cognitive function in the elderly (Ershler and Keller 2000; Cesari et al. 2004a,b; Ikeda 2003; Stocker and Keaney 2004).

Preliminary data indicate that the rate of aging at multiple levels, from subcellular organelles to social behavior, is largely synchronic, suggesting the existence of a single underlying mechanism. Consistent with this view, recent data suggest that a subset of older individuals has greater biological instability than their same age-peers and are, therefore, highly susceptible to multiple diseases and their functional consequences (Fried et al. 2004). These observations have led to the hypothesis that, in this particular group of persons, mechanisms that underlie aging processes are somehow accelerated and/or anticipated, and that age-related diseases and the multifaceted aspects of the aging process might share a common pathway.

---

[1] Clinical Research Branch, National Institute on Aging, Baltimore, MD, USA
[2] INRCA, Florence, Italy

Carey et al.
Longevity and Frailty

Geriatricians have proposed that older persons who are highly susceptible to disease and functional decline are affected by the "frailty syndrome," a relatively new clinical entity currently defined as "loss of functional reserve and resistance to stressors, resulting from the decline of biological stability across multiple physiological systems, associated with high risk of multiple adverse health outcomes" (Fried et al. 2001, 2004; Walston and Fried 1999).

## The conceptualization of frailty

Within the past five years, a frailty phenotype has been proposed and operationalized as the presence of at least three of the following five conditions: unintentional weight loss, poor grip strength, slow gait speed, feelings of exhaustion and low physical activity, suggesting that energy intake, distribution and expenditure are key features of the pathogenesis of frailty (Fried et al. 2001). It has been shown that older persons who meet the above criteria for frailty have an increased risk of hospitalization, falls, difficulty performing activities of daily living and death over three years of follow-up (Fried et al. 2001). Additionally, such persons exhibit a greater susceptibility to clinically evident and subclinical chronic diseases, particularly cardiovascular disease (Newman et al. 2001).

Identifying older persons affected by the frailty syndrome is an important initial step toward establishing new approaches to prevention and treatment. The availability of a working operational definition permits comparison of outcomes across different studies and opens the road to the design and conduct of clinical trials in this complex population (Ferrucci et al. 2004). Further advances in the clinical approach to frailty will require a better understanding of its intrinsic causes, pathophysiology and consequences.

According to current views, the frailty syndrome results from dysfunction in the physiological mechanisms that both maintain a stable homeostasis and re-establish homeostatic equilibrium after a destabilizing event occurs, in single cells as well as in the whole organism. It has been hypothesized that dysfunction in one or more of these mechanisms may be present well before signs and symptoms become clinically manifest in the form of a disease, impairment or functional limitation.

Operationally, the homeostatic system, a highly integrated functional network, encompasses multiple elements, including hormones, the immune response, the autonomic nervous system, and an intracellular energy production and distribution system (Girouard et al. 2003; Seeematter et al. 2004). Current research suggests that the intracellular energy production and distribution system is the weakest link of the network, primarily due to the role played by oxidative stress. Both very old and frail persons exhibit loss of effectiveness of these regulatory subsystems. A major consequence of this dysregulation is the inability of the regional distribution and production to adapt to extreme changes in the environment. Figure 1 illustrates this concept.

On the extreme left of the model depicted in Figure 1 lie the two main sources of energy that the organism acquires from the environment: dietary nutrients and oxygen. On the right, are the main sources of energy use, namely, physical

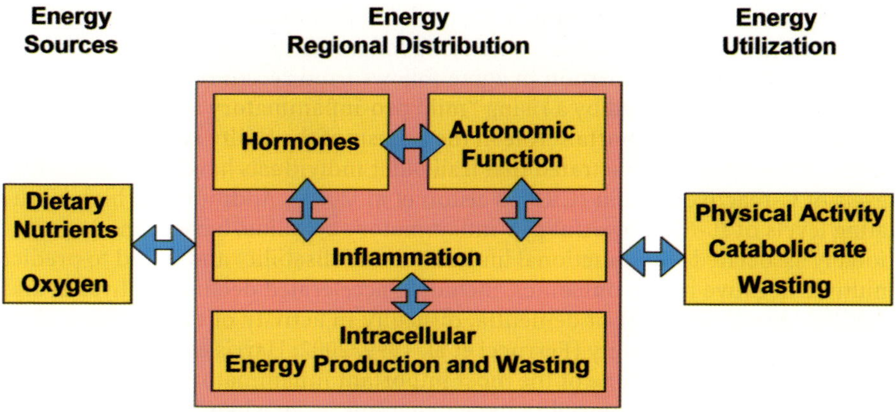


**Fig. 1.** Body energy delivery regulatory system

activity basal metabolic rate/maintainance. In the middle are all the physiological mechanisms and systems that maintain homeostasis in response to continual changes in the internal and external environment. In the overall picture, these systems 1) shift the production, delivery and utilization of energy from specific cells to other cells, as an adaptation response to current or expected future energy requirements; 2) maintain the concentration of nutrients within a specific range; 3) eliminate or reduce the concentration of potentially toxic waste products; 4) maintain an adequate production of signaling molecules; and 5) establish a hierarchy among the biological parameters, so that under stressful conditions, specific goals take priority over others. The elements of this network include 1) the intracellular system of energy production and delivery, including removal of waste products and toxic derivatives, in particular the oxidative stress/antioxidants system; 2) hormones, particularly those that directly regulate metabolic pathways; 3) immune function, including both immunologic cells and soluble immune mediators; and 4) the autonomic nervous system. Researchers have suggested that these physiological systems function in perfect and efficient harmony in young and middle-age adults but show progressive discord in late life. Accordingly, several lines of evidence indicate that hormones, byproducts of oxidative stress, inflammation and autonomic nervous system dysfunction play important roles in promoting disease states that are highly prevalent and frequent causes of functional incapacities in older persons (Girouard et al. 2003; Seematter et al. 2004; Genova et al. 2004; Lane 2003).

Researchers have proposed that the "secret" to perfect integration among regulatory systems involves the degree of complexity within each system and the set of rules that control the integration between systems. Consequently, aging can be interpreted as a reduction in complexity and a tendency to produce stereotypical responses to different stressors ( Lipsitz et al. 1992).

In the last few years, inflammation has become a major focus of research on the physiological basis of frailty. The recent accessibility of reliable and affordable tests that can measure large numbers of soluble inflammatory markers explains in part the growing enthusiasm for studying inflammation. Additionally, wide interest in studying inflammation in aging follows from recent research indicating that aging is characterized by a rising "mild pro-inflammatory state" and that inflammation plays an important role in the genesis of the frailty syndrome. In particular, it has been demonstrated that frail older individuals have high circulating levels of C-reactive protein (CRP; Walston et al. 2002). Additionally, high circulating levels of IL-6, a powerful pro-inflammatory cytokine, have been cross-sectionally associated with functional limitations and disability and found to predict multiple negative health outcomes, including accelerated decline of physical and cognitive function, onset of dementia, difficulty in activity of daily living (ADL) performance, and mortality (Ferrucci et al. 1999, 2002; Harris et al. 1999; Weaver et al. 2002). TNF-alpha, one of the most important inflammatory markers, is one of the few predictors of mortality in centenarians, even when the analysis is adjusted for disability and dementia (Bruunsgaard et al. 2003). Inflammation is also related to the five physiological domains included in the most commonly used operational definition of frailty. Inflammatory markers are cross-sectionally associated with low muscle strength, poor lower extremity performance, sedentary state, loss of appetite, inadequate nutrition and depressive symptoms (Cesari et al. 2004a; Morley 2001; Reuben et al. 2003; Penninx et al. 2003). High circulating levels of IL-6 predict an accelerated decline of physical performance, which is completely explained by the detrimental effect of IL-6 on muscle strength (Ferrucci et al. 2002). In addition, there is strong evidence that inflammation modulates the biological activity of several hormones, including insulin, IGF-1, and testosterone (Barbieri et al. 2003; Cappola et al. 2003; Ferrucci and Guralnk 2003). Together, these findings indicate that the aging process may be mediated by substantial up-regulation of the inflammatory response.

Is inflammation, therefore, the primary cause of the frailty syndrome? Although this question remains open, we believe that an affirmative answer is unlikely. By its intrinsic nature, inflammation is a response to a stress and not a primary, spontaneous process. Also, studies conducted in small clinical populations suggest that the inflammatory response to bacteria, vaccines and other extraneous antigens is substantially maintained over the aging process, although in older compared to younger persons, inflammation remains high for a longer time-period, indicating a primary impairment in the mechanisms that extinguish the inflammatory response when it is no longer required (Bruunsgaard et al. 1999). In our view, oxidative stress, rather than inflammation, is at the "core" of frailty. Unfortunately, the measures of oxidative stress available for use in humans are complex, expensive, and not very reliable. Consequently, evidence supporting the "oxidative stress" hypothesis of aging is currently limited.

## Oxidative stress causes an inflammatory response

Pre-clinical studies have shown that cardiovascular risk factors and cardiovascular morbidity are associated with severe oxidative stress and low circulating levels of antioxidants, suggesting that oxidative stress and inflammation may be

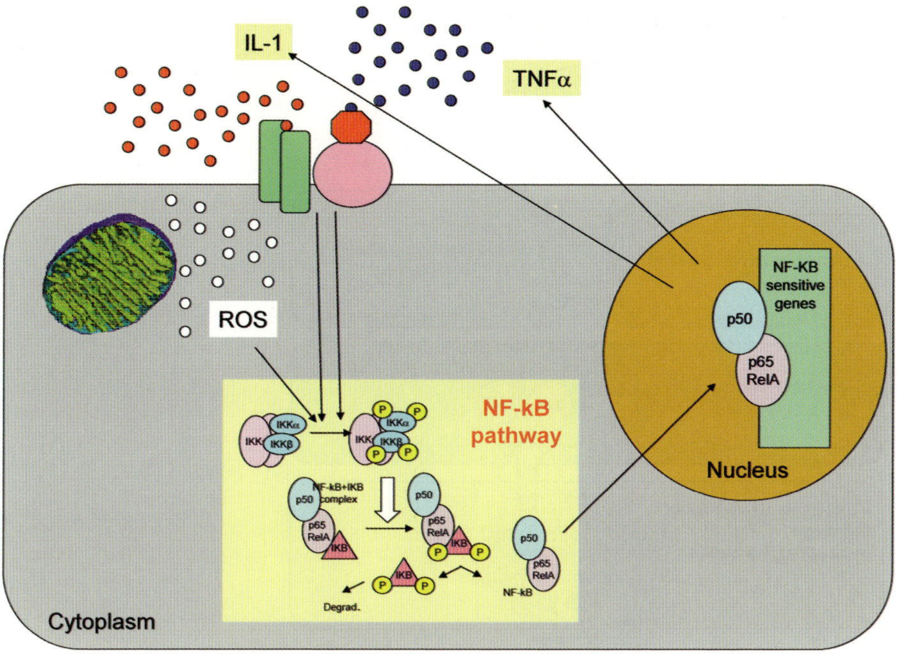


**Fig. 2.** Intracellular mechanisms linking oxidative stress and cytokines production

two sides of the same coin (Lane 2003). In particular, oxidative stress is known to stimulate production of several cytokines (including IL-6) via activation of the NF-kB pathway (May and Ghosh 1998; Fig. 2). According to this view, inflammation might be an epiphenomenon of intracellular modifications induced by oxidative stress. Age-related decline in the efficiency of the respiratory chain may lead to the production of excessive quantities of free radicals that, through continuous activation of the NF-kB pathway, lead to a chronic, mild inflammatory state.

Inflammation constitutes the signaling pathway that connects the cell environment to cells in the same and other tissues, interacts with the production and biological activity of several hormones, modulates the effectiveness and efficacy of autonomic nervous system reflexes and, in turn, amplifies the inflammatory response (Fig. 3). For example, with an acute exposure to an infectious organism, there is insufficient time and energy to build new muscle, so cytokines inhibit production and activity of IGF-1. By delaying this activity to a more appropriate time, the organism can then divert the energy this would have required and use it to deal with the stressor. In an acute situation, this strategy is essential for building defense mechanisms that can eliminate the threat of an external attack and simultaneously protect the integrity of the organism. However, if there is no attacker to be eliminated and the inflammatory state is maintained by an intrinsic mitochondrial dysfunction, the persistence of the "emergency" state (without any true emergency) is deleterious and may lead to degenerative processes

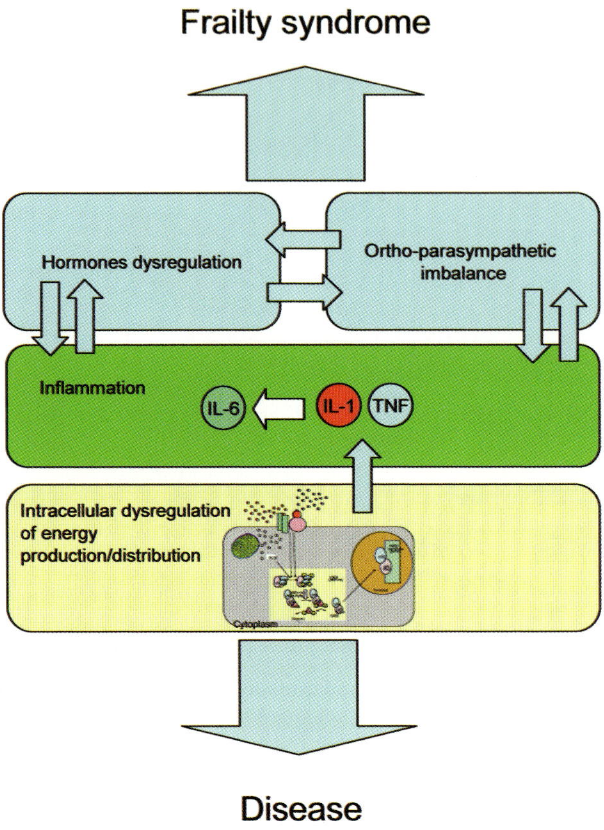


**Fig. 3.** Hypothesized common pathogenesis of frailty syndrome and age-related diseases

and disease initiation. In the context of this theory, researchers have proposed a trade-off between the efficiency of inflammation as a defense against infections and uncontrolled inflammation as a cause of age-related frailty. Interestingly, the only intervention that has been shown to reduce the risk of disability is physical activity, which has consistently shown a strong effect in reducing oxidative stress, increasing the quantity and efficiency of antioxidant barriers, and reducing circulating levels of the main inflammatory markers. Unfortunately, beyond exercise, no other intervention is known to reduce the rate of oxidative stress. Currently available pharmacological approaches to control inflammation are imprecise because they do not impact on selected pathways. To successfully treat frailty we need to learn how to more subtly modulate the immune system and the stress response than we know at present. We need to make a connection between the different aspects of aging and frailty at the molecular, cellular, tissue, physiological and functional levels, and introduce these parallel perspectives in newly designed observational studies. Finally, we need to develop the techniques and experience needed to successfully conduct clinical trials in frail older persons.

## References

Barbieri M, Ferrucci L, Ragno E, Corsi A, Bandinelli S, Bonafe M, Olivieri F, Giovagnetti S, Franceschi C, Guralnik JM, Paolisso G (2003) Chronic inflammation and the effect of IGF-I on muscle strength and power in older persons. Am J Physiol Endocrinol Metab 284:E481-487.

Bruunsgaard H, Skinhoj P, Qvist J, Pedersen BK (1999) Elderly humans show prolonged in vivo inflammatory activity during pneumococcal infections. J Infect Dis 180:551-554.

Bruunsgaard H, Andersen-Ranberg K, Hjelmborg JB, Pedersen BK, Jeune B (2003) Elevated levels of tumor necrosis factor alpha and mortality in centenarians. Am J Med 115:278-283.

Cappola AR, Xue QL, Ferrucci L, Guralnik JM, Volpato S, Fried LP (2003) Insulin-like growth factor I and interleukin-6 contribute synergistically to disability and mortality in older women. J Clin Endocrinol Metab 88:2019-2025.

Cesari M, Penninx BW, Pahor M, Lauretani F, Corsi AM, Rhys Williams G, Guralnik JM, Ferrucci L (2004) Inflammatory markers and physical performance in older persons: the InCHIANTI study. J Gerontol A Biol Sci Med Sci 59:242-248.

Cesari M, Pahor M, Bartali B, Cherubini A, Penninx BW, Williams GR, Atkinson H, Martin A, Guralnik JM, Ferrucci L (2004) Antioxidants and physical performance in elderly persons: the Invecchiare in Chianti (InCHIANTI) study. Am J Clin Nutr 79:289-294.

Di Carlo A, Baldereschi M, Amaducci L, Maggi S, Grigoletto F, Scarlato G, Inzitari D. (2000) Cognitive impairment without dementia in older people: prevalence, vascular risk factors, impact on disability. The Italian Longitudinal Study on Aging. J Am Geriatr Soc 48:775-782.

Ershler WB, Keller ET (2000) Age-associated increased interleukin-6 gene expression, late-life diseases, and frailty. Annu Rev Med 51:245-270.

Ferrucci L, Guralnik JM (2003) Inflammation, hormones, and body composition at a crossroad. Am J Med 115:501-502.

Ferrucci L, Harris TB, Guralnik JM, Tracy RP, Corti MC, Cohen HJ, Penninx B, Pahor M, Wallace R, Havlik RJ (1999) Serum IL-6 level and the development of disability in older persons. J Am Geriatr Soc 47:639-646.

Ferrucci L, Penninx BW, Volpato S, Harris TB, Bandeen-Roche K, Balfour J, Leveille SG, Fried LP, Guralnik JM (2002) Change in muscle strength explains accelerated decline of physical function in older women with high interleukin-6 serum levels. J Am Geriatr Soc 50:1947-1954.

Ferrucci L, Guralnik JM, Studenski S, Fried LP, Cutler GB, Jr., Walston JD (2003) Designing randomized, controlled trials aimed at preventing or delaying functional decline and disability in frail, older persons: a consensus report. J Am Geriatr Soc 52:625-634.

Fried LP, Tangen CM, Walston J, Newman AB, Hirsch C, Gottdiener J, Seeman T, Tracy R, Kop WJ, Burke G, McBurnie MA (2001) Frailty in older adults: evidence for a phenotype. J Gerontol A Biol Sci Med Sci 56:M146-156.

Fried LP, Ferrucci L, Darer J, Williamson JD, Anderson G (2004) Untangling the concepts of disability, frailty, and comorbidity: implications for improved targeting and care. J Gerontol A Biol Sci Med Sci 59:255-263.

Genova ML, Pich MM, Bernacchia A, Bernacchia A, Bianchi C, Biondi A, Bovina A, Falasca AI, Formiggini G, Castelli GP, Lenaz G (2004) The mitochondrial production of reactive oxygen species in relation to aging and pathology. Ann NY Acad Sci 1011:86-100.

Girouard H, Chulak C, LeJossec M, Lamontagne D, de Champlain J (2003) Chronic antioxidant treatment improves sympathetic functions and beta-adrenergic pathway in the spontaneously hypertensive rats. J Hypertens 21:179-188.

Harris TB, Ferrucci L, Tracy RP, Corti MC, Wacholder S, Ettinger WH Jr, Heimovitz H, Cohen HJ, Wallace R (1999) Associations of elevated interleukin-6 and C-reactive protein levels with mortality in the elderly. Am J Med 106:506-512.

Ikeda U (2003) Inflammation and coronary artery disease. Curr Vasc Pharmacol 1:65-70.

Lane N (2003) A unifying view of ageing and disease: the double-agent theory. J Theor Biol 225:531-540.

Lipsitz LA, Goldberger AL (1992) Loss of 'complexity' and aging. Potential applications of fractals and chaos theory to senescence. JAMA 267:1806-1809.

May MJ, Ghosh S (1998) Signal transduction through NF-kappa B. Immunol Today 19:80-88

Morley JE (2001) Decreased food intake with aging. J Gerontol A Biol Sci Med Sci 56 Spec No 2:81-88.

Newman AB, Gottdiener JS, McBurnie MA, Hirsch CH, Kop WJ, Tracy R, Walston JD, Fried LP (2001) Associations of subclinical cardiovascular disease with frailty. J Gerontol A Biol Sci Med Sci 56:M158-166.

Penninx BW, Kritchevsky SB, Yaffe K, Newman AB, Simonsick EM, Rubin S, Ferrucci L, Harris T, Pahor M(2003) Inflammatory markers and depressed mood in older persons: results from the Health, Aging and Body Composition study. Biol Psychiat 54:566-572.

Reuben DB, Judd-Hamilton L, Harris TB, Seeman TE (2003) The associations between physical activity and inflammatory markers in high-functioning older persons: MacArthur Studies of Successful Aging. J Am Geriatr Soc 51:1125-1130.

Seematter G, Binnert C, Martin JL, Tappy L (2004) Relationship between stress, inflammation and metabolism. Curr Opin Clin Nutr Metab Care 7:169-173.

Stocker R, Keaney JF, Jr. (2004) Role of oxidative modifications in atherosclerosis. Physiol Rev 84:1381-1478.

Vaupel JW, Carey JR, Christensen K, Johnson TE, Yashin AI, Holm NV, Iachine IA, Kannisto V, Khazaeli AA, Liedo P, Longo VD, Zeng Y, Manton KG, Curtsinger JW (1998) Biodemographic trajectories of longevity. Science. 280:855-860.

Walston J, Fried LP (1999) Frailty and the older man. Med Clin North Am 83:1173-1194.

Walston J, McBurnie MA, Newman A, Tracy RP, Kop WJ, Hirsch CH, Gottdiener J, Fried LP (2002) Frailty and activation of the inflammation and coagulation systems with and without clinical comorbidities: results from the Cardiovascular Health Study. Arch Intern Med 162:2333-2341.

Weaver JD, Huang MH, Albert M, Harris T, Rowe JW, Seeman TE (2002) Interleukin-6 and risk of cognitive decline: MacArthur studies of successful aging. Neurology 59:371-378.

# Early Life Conditions Affect Historical Change in Old-Age Mortality

*Eileen M. Crimmins*[1] *and Caleb E. Finch*[1]

## Summary

Adult life expectancy has progressively increased over the past 150 years, equivalent to one year added per four years of historical time in high life-expectancy populations. This amazing decline of mortality at all adult ages is attributed to environmental and technological advances. Explanations of the decline in long-term mortality typically are seated in terms of period or historical factors, to the neglect of cohort or life cycle factors. From associations between the early and later age mortality for birth cohorts, we argue that historical reduction in lifetime exposure to infectious diseases and other sources of inflammation is a major cause of the decline in old age mortality.

## Introduction

Researchers have long noted the association between early and later age mortality. In 1934, Kermack et al. noticed a pattern of historical changes in birth cohorts from England and Sweden: as the mortality levels in early life improved in successive historical cohorts, the adult survivors in those cohorts also had lower mortality. They hypothesized that maternal health and child health were major determinants of health at later ages, i.e., the mortality characteristics of a cohort persisted throughout its life span. In 1956, Jones further developed links between lower cohort mortality at younger and older ages in Swedish data, concluding that recent cohorts had similar mortality slopes across the adult ages, but mortality curves were displaced to lower values. Jones characterized "the physiological age of each new generation as remaining more youthful at the same chronological age." We have designated this imprint of early life as "the cohort morbidity phenotype" (Finch and Crimmins 2004). In this paper we provide further evidence of the cohort morbidity phenotype and discuss its implications for understanding historical mortality change.

[1] Andrus Gerontology Center, University of Southern California, 3715 McClintock Avenue, Los Angeles, CA 90089-0191, USA

Carey et al.
Longevity and Frailty

## Mortality Across the Age Range

The links between mortality at younger and older ages have been confirmed by a number of contemporary researchers (Azbel 2002; Davey Smith and Ben-Shlomo 1997; Yashin et al. 2002); for example, Azbel (2002) showed a high correlation between mortality before 20 and later adult mortality in Swedish cohorts. We have shown that, in Sweden cohorts spanning 150 years, mortality for successive cohorts is lower at each age across the age range (Fig. 1a). We have also noted that the link between old-age and young-age mortality is only clear when mortality is displayed in a cohort, as opposed to a period, format (Finch and Crimmins 2004). The age-specific mortality curves in period format for Sweden do not show the same pattern of successively lower mortality at the older ages (Fig. 1b).

Age-specific mortality at adult ages is well known to be related as specified by the Gompertz curve, in which the mortality rate at adult age ($x$) is a function of background mortality ($a$, age invariant constant) and exponentially increasing mortality with a monotonic mortality slope, $b$ (Jones 1956; Strehler 1960):

$$\text{In}[m(x)] = a + bx \qquad \text{(Eq. 1)}$$

While the theory underlying the Gompertz model is generally a cohort or life cycle theory, the curve has been derived from observations of period data. We note that examination of the period and cohort data formulations has implications for generalizations about the slope of mortality increase with age. While both these sets of Swedish mortality curves approximate the Gompertz model of mortality, slopes at adult ages before 60 are shallower and vary more than at later ages, particularly in earlier times, such that historical populations often deviate widely from the monotonic Gompertz model. Moreover, there is a greater convergence of curves at later ages in periods than in cohorts.

The Gompertz model is the basis for the "Strehler- Mildvan general theory of mortality" (Strehler and Mildvan 1960). This model predicts an inverse correlation between ln($a$) values extrapolated to birth and Gompertz slopes ($b$) at later ages, based on their observations of selected mid-20th century period mortality curves for populations. According to this model, high early mortality is associated with slower mortality accelerations among adults; that is, higher early mortality slows the rate of demographic aging. However, Yashin et al. (2002) showed that recent cohorts diverge from Strehler-Mildvan. Moreover, Gavrilov and Gravilova (2003) argue that the Strehler-Mildvan theory is flawed because, as an extrapolation, it neglects true background mortality. Further, we observe that the higher early adult mortality in earlier times reduces the overall slope of mortality curves (Fig.1 a,b), which inevitably makes more recent mortality slopes steeper, but without recourse to Strehler-Mildvan. In sum, despite their divergences about levels and slopes, these analyses agree that early mortality importantly influences later mortality.

The cohort mortality curves for the entire age range for five cohorts born from 1751 to 1940 (with extrapolated data for the last cohort) illustrate how the powerful cohort effects have downshifted age-specific mortality curves so that mortality at any given age is successively lower in cohorts after 1751 (Fig. 1a). The impor-

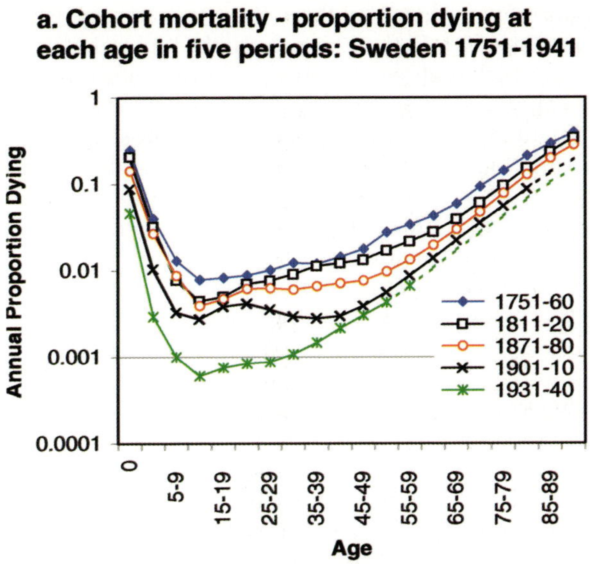


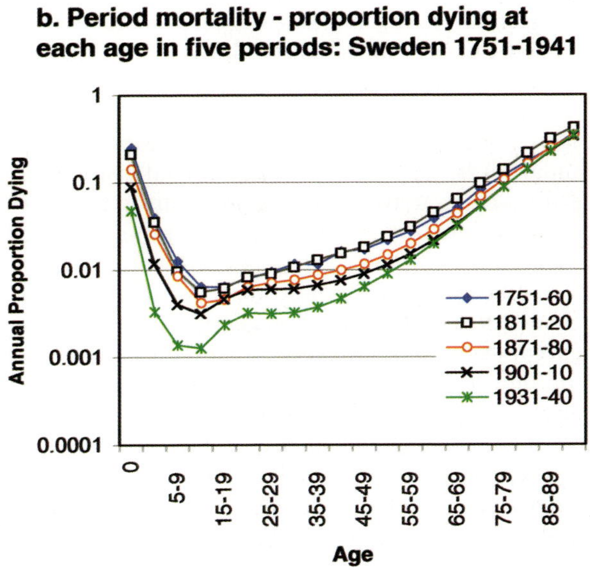


**Fig. 1.** Mortality over the life span. **a** Cohort mortality – proportion dying at each age in five periods: Sweden 1751–1941 **b** Period mortality – proportion dying at each age in five periods: Sweden 1751–1941 (Source: Berkeley Mortality Data Base) Mortality is estimated for the later years of the last cohort assuming that mortality at adjacent age groups has a similar relationship to that in the next earlier cohort. Source: Berkeley Mortality Data Base. (Finch and Crimmins 2004)

tance of this shift in cohort mortality is shown by the shift of the later age when each cohort reaches a mortality risk of 0.1. In the 1751 cohort, the 0.1 level of mortality occurred at age 73.4 years, which is about 10 years earlier than our estimate (84 years) for the 1931-1940 cohort. The cohort–period difference between the age patterns of mortality is evident by comparing the period and cohort mortality schedules for the same dates (Fig. 1a,b). The Gompertz slopes do not differ after 1871 for cohorts, consistent with Yashin et al. (2002). Because these rapid changes in mortality occurred in Sweden during a time of negligible immigration, it seems unlikely that changes in cohort mortality are due to changes in genetic polymorphisms or new genotypes, but rather to environmental imprinting, at some level. We argue that inflammatory processes provide such a mechanism.

## Life Expectancy Change Across Age and Time

In this section we document that historical mortality decline among the young and old began in the same cohorts. We continue to use Sweden as an example, because of availability of reliable and valid data over a long period of time. We examine long-term trends from 1751 through 2001 in life expectancy at birth ($e_0$), from birth to age 70 ($e_{0\text{-}70}$), and at age 70 ($e_{70}$). Reductions in mortality at the older ages should lag behind reductions in the younger ages. Four periods of increased life expectancy at birth in Sweden can be delineated: Period I (1751-1790), no real change (maybe even decrease) in life expectancy (the pre-modern norm); Period II (1791-1870), slow increase; Period III (1871-1950), very rapid increase; and Period IV, (1951-2000), slower increase. Changes in total life expectancy at birth and up to age 70 are similar in the first three periods. The intensity of the decrease in infectious disease also differs across these periods. During Period II, smallpox vaccination was introduced into Sweden and clean water was increased (Bengtsson and Lindstrom 2000; Fridlizius 1989). Period III represented the control of infections gained with the understanding of the germ theory and development of public health practices and, eventually, antibiotics. Period IV, with slower increases in life expectancy except at the older ages, was marked by the virtual elimination of early deaths from infectious conditions and increasing life expectancy before old age, with diseases of aging becoming predominant.

Life expectancy in old age ($e_{70}$) shows a definite lag behind increases of $e_0$ and $e_{0\text{-}70}$. There is no sustained increase of $e_{70}$ until Period III, and this increase is modest relative to Period IV. This lag is consistent with the cohort morbidity phenotype determined by environmental conditions early in the life span.

## Environmental explanations of cohort morbidity and mortality

Reduction of infectious disease is recognized as the main factor in improved cohort survival (Elo and Preston 1992; Floud et al. 1990; Riley 2001). Long before modern medicine (antibiotics, comprehensive vaccination, vascular surgery), public health innovations reduced exposure to infections. This reduction was accomplished through programs of vaccinations and improvement of water supplies. With development of modern means of sanitation, exposure to infection was markedly reduced. Increased income also allowed lower density housing and sufficient and clean clothing. Access to a balanced diet of uncontaminated food throughout the year improved resistance to infection.

Early life infections are strongly associated with later morbidity, including cardiovascular and respiratory disease, cancer, and diabetes. A classic example is rheumatic heart disease, which increases adult morbidity when heart valves are damaged during childhood streptococcal infections. Other post-infection sequelae include impaired immune responses and lowered resistance, even if pathogens are attenuated; for example, early respiratory infections are associated with later lung impairments (Shaheen et al. 1994). Among U.S. Civil War veterans, infectious disease in early adulthood was associated with heart and respiratory problems after age 50 (Costa 2000). Adult cardiovascular disease in the U.S from 1961-71 is also associated with infant diarrhea and enteritis (Buck and Simpson, 1982). Among people currently in their 50s, major childhood illness is associated with 15% more cardiovascular conditions and 100% more cancer and chronic lung conditions (Blackwell et al. 2001). Costa has estimated that the decline in infectious diseases may explain 11- 24% of the decline of both morbid and mortal conditions at age 60-74 over most of the 20$^{th}$ Century (Costa 2000).

We have suggested that a reduction in lifelong levels of inflammation accompanied this reduction in infectious disease, and this lower level of inflammation is a vital link between infection in early life and health in late life (Finch and Crimmins 2004). The inflammatory acute phase response to infection is essential but it may promote the development of disease later in life. While inflammatory responses in historical populations cannot be measured, there is ample evidence of the relationship of infection and inflammation. C-reactive protein (CRP), an acute-phase inflammatory protein that mediates the clearance of invading bacteria, is elevated in chronic infectious diseases that were common in high mortality populations. For example, active tuberculosis (TB) is associated with high CRP (Lawn et al. 2000), as is diarrhea (Cadwgan et al. 2000). Growing evidence links earlier infections to higher levels of inflammation. Increasing evidence links chronically high levels of inflammation to multiple diseases of aging (Finch and Crimmins 2004).

Reduced levels of infection occurring with the increase in life expectancy were accompanied by reductions in infectious conditions that are included as sources of inflammation in Table 1. Additional improvements in other environmental inflammogens undoubtedly also came about because of changes in the non-infectious environment accompanying income growth. Changes in living and workplace conditions and reductions in traumatic injuries also have contributed to hypothesized societal levels of inflammation. The increase of inflammation among those engaging in strenuous exercise (Siegel et al. 2001) implies another inflammatory source in those who suffer the relentless physical labor that is common in disadvantaged populations.

**Table 1.** Inflammatory factors that improved in populations with increased life expectancy

| Inflammatory environment | | | Nutrition-infection interactions |
|---|---|---|---|
| Infections | Non-infectious environment<br>Chemical-physical | <br>Social-lifestyle | |
| Cholera | Aerosolst | Disturbed sleep | Micronutrient deficits |
| *H. pylori* | Dust, | crowding, noise | impair growth and |
| Influenza | fecal endotoxins, | Emotional stress | immune functions |
| Measles | smoke | Physical stress | |
| Parasites | Chemical pollutants | and trauma | Gut infections reduce |
| Crabs, malaria, | Lead, mercury, $SO_2$ | Endless physical labor, | nutrient availability |
| worms | Contaminated food | serial pregnancy, | |
| Periodontal disease | Noise | social violence | Spoiled food |
| Smallpox | Temperature extremes | | |
| Syphilis | | | |
| Typhus | | | |
| Tuberculosis | | | |

## Conclusions

Major factors that have improved childhood health and survival by reducing infectious disease and chronic inflammatory conditions include improved public health and personal hygiene, developments in dentistry and medicine, reduced home crowding and bed sharing, reduced aerosols, and availability of a balanced diet throughout the year (Table 1). The progressive improvements in human mortality, which began before 1800, have therefore not only improved childhood health but also reduced the inflammatory status throughout life. This view radically departs from assumptions that infectious causes of childhood diseases have little to do with the major diseases of aging, chiefly vascular disease, cancer, and Alzheimer's disease, which are not infectious *between* adults.

The stability of cohort mortality slopes, despite the remarkable downshift in overall mortality, implies that future increases in life expectancy from reduced inflammatory causes may be small, because early age mortality *must* approach a lower limit. A major question is the effect of childhood infections on host defense systems that interact with major causes of adult mortality during aging. Longitudinal blood samples may become available to allow tracking of CRP and other inflammatory markers from birth throughout the life span. During normal aging in many organs, many of the same inflammatory genes are induced in the absence of specific pathology; moreover, the age changes can be modulated by diet (Wilson et al. 2002). We do not know how inflammatory processes of aging interact with specific diseases (vascular disease, some cancers, and Alzheimer's disease) that have inflammatory mechanisms. Findings from many fields suggest that inflammatory processes that affect outcomes of aging can be kindled or quenched by extrinsic infections, inflammatory stimuli, and nutrition. A new theory of human health in life history could emerge from a fuller accounting of inflammatory exposures.

## References

Azbel MY (2002) An exact law can test biological theories of mortality. Exp Gerontol 37: 859-869.

Bengtsson T, Lindstrom M (2000) Childhood misery and disease in later life: The effects on mortality in old age of hazards experienced in early life, southern Sweden, 1760-1894. Pop Stud 54: 263-277.

Blackwell DL, Hayward MD, Crimmins EM (2001) Does childhood health affect chronic morbidity in later life? Soc Sci Med 52: 1269-84.

Buck C, Simpson, H (1982) Infant diarrhoea and subsequent mortality from heart disease and cancer. J Epidemiol Commun Health 36: 27-30.

Cadwgan AM, Watson WA, Laing RB, MacKenzie AR, Smith CC, Douglas JG (2000) Presenting clinical features and C-reactive protein in the prediction of a positive stool culture in patients with diarrhoea. J Infect 41: 159-61.

Costa DL (2000) Understanding the twentieth century decline in chronic conditions among older men. Demography 37:53-62.

Davey Smith G, Ben-Shlomo Y (1997) Geographical and social class differences in stroke mortality - the influence of early-life factors: comment on papers by Maheswaran and colleagues. J Epidemiol Commun Health 51: 134-137.

Elo TI, Preston HS (1992) Effects of early-life conditions on adult mortality: A review. Pop Index 58:86-212.

Finch CE, Crimmins EM (2004) Inflammatory exposure and historical changes in human lifespans. Science 305: 1736-1739.

Floud R, Wachter K, Gregory A (1990) Height, health, and history. In: Laslett P, Schofeld R,Wrigley, EA, Smith DS, (eds) Cambridge studies in population, economy, and society in past time. Cambridge University Press, New York, Vol. 9.

Fridlizius G (1989) The deformation of cohorts: nineteenth century mortality decline in a generational perspective. Scand Econ Hist Rev 37: 3-17.

Gavrilov LA, Gavrilova NS (2003) The quest for a general theory of aging and longevity. http//sageke.sciencemag.org/cgi/content/full/2003/28/re5.

Jones HB (1956) Life span and age-specific death rate. A special consideration of the aging Ppocess, disease, and life expectancy. Adv Biol Med Phys 4: 281-337.

Kermack WO, McKendrick AG, McKinlay PL (1934) Death-rates in Great Britain and Sweden. Lancet i:698-703.

Lawn SD, Obeng J, Acheampong JW, Griffin GE (2000) Resolution of the acute-phase response in West African patients receiving treatment for pulmonary tuberculosis. Int J Tuberc Lung Dis 4: 340-4.

Oeppen J, Vaupel JW (2002) Broken limits to life expectancy. Science 296: 1029-1031.

Riley JC (2001) Rising life expectancy: A global history. Cambridge: Cambridge University Press.

Shaheen SO,Barker DJ, Shiell AW, Crocker FJ, Wield GA, Holgate ST (1994) The relationship between pneumonia in early childhood and impaired lung function in late adult life. Am J Resp Crit Care Med 149: 616-619.

Siegel AJ, Stec JJ, Lipinska I, Van Cott EM, Lewandrowski KB, Ridker PM, Tofler GH (2001) Effect of marathon running on inflammatory and hemostatic markers. Am J Cardiol 88: 918-20.

Strehler BL, Mildvan AS (1960) General theory of mortality and aging. Science 132: 14-21.

Wilson CJ, Finch CE, Cohen HJ (2002) Cytokines and Cognition: The case for A Head-to-Toe Inflammation Paradigm. J Am Ger Soc 50: 2041-2056

Yashin AI, Begun AS, Boiko SI, Ukraintseva SV, Oeppen J (2002) New age patterns of survival improvement in Sweden: do they characterize changes in individual aging? Mech Aging Devel 123: 637-647.

# Aging, Frailty, and the Compression of Morbidity: Definite Progress

*James F. Fries*[1]

## Summary

Frailty, the loss of physiologic organ reserve with age, and chronic illness, which may accelerate the development of frailty in one or more than one body system, become the dominant determinants of ill-health in those who escape the hazards of early and mid-life. The Compression of Morbidity paradigm holds that if the average age at first infirmity, disability, or other morbidity is postponed, and if this postponement is greater than increases in life expectancy, then average cumulative lifetime morbidity will decrease, squeezed between a later onset and the time of death. The National Long-Term Care Survey, the National Health Interview Survey, and other data from the United States and some other developed countries now document declining disability trends beginning around 1982 and accelerating more recently. The decline in disability is about 2% per year, contrasted with a decline in mortality rates of about 1% a year, documenting compression of morbidity in the United States at the population level. Longitudinal studies now link good health risk status with long-term reductions in cumulative lifetime disability; those with few behavioral health risks have only one-fourth the disability of those who have more risk factors, and the onset of disability in those with good health habits is postponed from 7 to 12 years, far more than any increases in longevity. Randomized controlled trials of health enhancement programs in senior populations have shown a reduction in health risks, improved health status, and decreased medical care utilization. Health policy initiatives now being undertaken have the promise of increasing and consolidating health gains for seniors under the umbrella paradigm of the Compression of Morbidity.

## Introduction

The Compression of Morbidity paradigm was presented as a hypothesis in 1980 (Fries 1980); it noted that the great majority of illness was chronic and occurred in later life and postulated that the lifetime burden of illness could be reduced if the onset of chronic illness could be postponed and if this postponement could be greater than increases in life expectancy. The concept is illustrated in Figure 1,

[1] From the Department of Medicine, Stanford University School of Medicine, Stanford, California. Address reprint requests to Dr. Fries at 1000 Welch Road, Suite 203, Palo Alto, CA 94304

Carey et al.
Longevity and Frailty

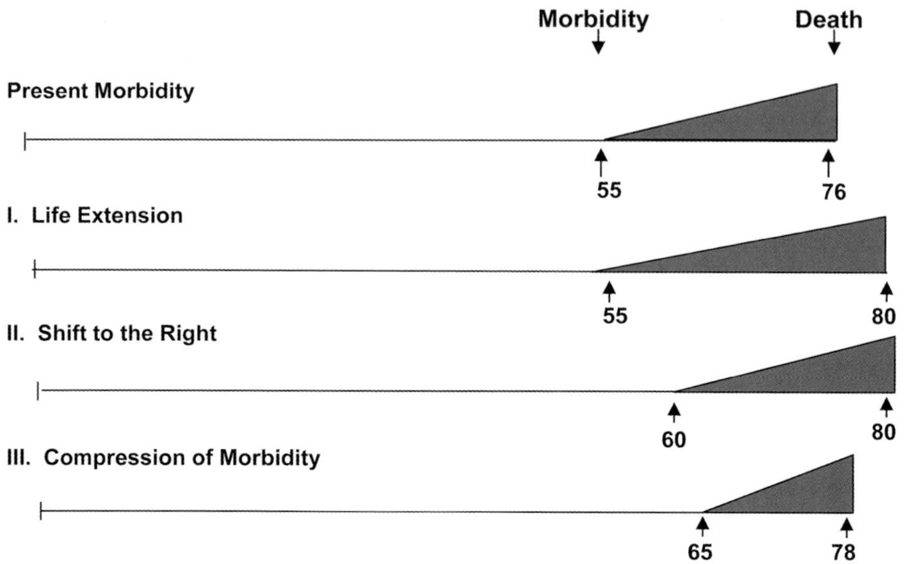


**Fig. 1.** Possible Scenarios for Future Morbidity and Longevity

where estimated present lifetime morbidity is portrayed along with three possible future scenarios: "life extension," "shift-to-the-right," and "compression of morbidity." The lines represent the length of life and the shaded triangle depicts lifetime morbidity. Two arrows are shown for each scenario: the left arrow represents the median age of onset of chronic morbidity and the right arrow the median age at death. Alternative health futures are determined by the relative movement of these arrows over time. If the arrows separate, there is more lifetime morbidity; if they come closer together, there is compression of morbidity. In each scenario some extension of life expectancy is envisioned, although this expectation is not inevitable. The illustrative use of age 55 years as the present age of onset of chronic morbidity is drawn from our data showing this to be the median age of detectable chronic disability (Bruce and Fries 2003).

Most demographers and health policy workers in 1980 felt that the "life extension" scenario was occurring and was the most likely, and most unfortunate, future for human health. As medical progress increasingly prolonged life, those extra months and years would be spent in poorer and poorer health. The process was termed the "failure of success"(Gruenberg 2003).

In contrast, the Compression of Morbidity represented a positive concept, with the ideal of a long life with a relatively short period of terminal decline, and it was initially sometimes portrayed as naively optimistic and perhaps a threat to the social preparation required to care for ever-larger senior populations in the future (Myers and Menton 1984; Verbrugge 1984). A problem in 1980 was that there were few data available on trends in morbidity; such data would have required serial population surveys that used similar methods and these were not available. There was not even an agreed definition of "morbidity" then, nor is there now. It seemed reasonable in 1980 to postulate that lifetime morbidity had been rising with the emergence of chronic illnesses, but it could be argued that this period was ending with declining incidences of major chronic illnesses, such as cardiovascular disease (Fries 1980).

The Compression of Morbidity paradigm focuses attention on the quality–of life over its quantity and considers morbidity as a lifetime, cumulative area-under-the-curve concept rather than a cross-sectional view at a particular point of time, such as a specific age. It suggests that the national burden of illness may be reduced by postponing the onset of infirmity. Thus, the national illness burden, which will increase with an increasing number of seniors in the population, may be offset, at least in part, by a lower average illness burden for the individual, with positive consequences for the health of the public and the stability of national health care systems.

This paper draws upon recent data from national surveys, observational longitudinal studies, and randomized controlled trials to bring together the present evidence for compression of morbidity in the United States and to outline the research agenda for the continued monitoring of trends in morbidity and disability.

Given appropriate data, the compression hypothesis can be tested using age-specific disability rates or cumulative lifetime disability as surrogates for the less easily defined "morbidity" rates. Trends in age-specific disability can then be compared with trends in age-specific mortality, and trends toward a postponed point of incident disability can be compared with trends toward a postponed age at death. If age-specific disability declines faster than age-specific mortality, then compression is established. Even better, if given serial cohorts of longitudinal data, trends in cumulative lifetime disability could be assessed. Further, if disability can be postponed by specific interventions (such as exercise, weight control, total joint replacement, influenza vaccination or smoking cessation) by more than projected increases in the length of life from these interventions, then a strategy for reduction in the national burden of illness by dissemination of such interventions would be mandated.

## Trends in Mortality

Since morbidity compression depends upon the relative trends in morbidity rates and in mortality rates, it is necessary first to examine trends in life expectancy. From 1980 to 1998, life expectancy (US data, both sexes combined) rose at a rate of 0.150 years per year, for an increase of 2.7 years, to 76.6 years, somewhat slower than in the two prior decades (Kranczer 1999). The more relevant number, however, is life expectancy from age 65 (or even 85), since this excludes the large effects of early life mortality. From age 65, life expectancy rose at a rate of only 0.066 per year, for an increase of 1.2 years over 18 years, to a life expectancy of 82.7 years; this is a slightly lower rate of increase than in prior decades. From age 85, life expectancy rose by only 0.017 years per year, for an increase of 0.3 years or only about four months over the past 18 years. Similar data are available in every developed nation (excepting most states of the former Soviet Union). If present trends continue, gains in average life expectancy above age 65 will remain modest in magnitude. However, because of larger birth cohorts and an increasing proportion of persons surviving to age 65, the absolute number of persons over 65 years of age will increase markedly.

Present trends will not continue indefinitely, moreover. Barring discovery and dissemination of a breakthrough in understanding of the basic science of aging, the rate of increase in human life expectancy to advanced ages will continue to slow. Constant decreases in mortality rates, about 1% a year, yield diminishing increases in terms of life expectancy over time because of the exponential mathematical relationship between the two statistics; the effect of constant mortality rate decreases yields smaller increments of life expectancy over time (Olshansky and Ault 1986). This can be seen with the "point of paradox," in which projected life expectancy from birth, rising more rapidly than projected life expectancy from age 65, intersects with the life expectancy from age 65 projection at life expectancy of 87.8 years in the year 2076, using current US data. Since life expectancy ages computed from birth cannot surpass life expectancy ages computed from advanced ages, present trends cannot continue indefinitely.

## Trends in Morbidity

Over the past two decades, we could have wished for a great natural experiment in the developed world in which preventive measures, which are most relevant to postponement of morbidity, had been broadly implemented. On a national basis, there could have been massive reductions in health risk factors such as cigarette smoking, obesity, and lack of exercise. Then, with emerging data on trends in disability, particularly from the National Long-Term Care Survey (NLTCS; Manton and Gu 2001) and the National Health Interview Survey (NHIS; Schoeni et al. 2001), we could have assessed the benefits from these changes against changes in mortality. Unfortunately, whereas smoking did decrease significantly in the US, obesity and the "metabolic syndrome" greatly increased in prevalence, and there has been a trend toward more sedentary lifestyles. Over the last two decades, therefore, lifestyle changes are not likely to have played a dominant causal role in the compression of morbidity.

However, compression of morbidity has been occurring, and at a relatively rapid rate. In the NLTCS data (Table 1), disability over age 65 decreased from 26.2% to 19.7% from 1982 to 1999, a decrease of approximately 2% per year and substantially greater than decreases in mortality rates, which declined at about 1% per year, their historical rate of decline over the past century (Cutler 2001). The decline was seen both in activities of daily living (ADL) disability and instrumental, more complex activities of daily living (IADL) disability. It has been argued that a decline in age-specific disability of 1.5% per year would be sufficient to maintain the solvency of the US Medicare Program for at least 70 years (Singer and Manton 1998). Moreover, the declines in disability found by the NLTCS have accelerated in the last five years of observation and have begun to be seen in minority as well as white sub-populations (Manton and Gu 2001). Data from the

**Table 1.** Population disability distribution National Long-term care survey disability and housing (%) (Adapted from Manton and Gu, 2001)

| | 1982 | 1984 | 1989 | 1994 | 1999 |
|---|---|---|---|---|---|
| Total % Disabled | 26.2 | 26.2 | 24.4 | 22.5 | 19.7 |
| Mild Disab (IADL) | 5.7 | 6.2 | 4.8 | 4.4 | 3.2 |
| Moderate Disab (1-2) | 6.9 | 7.0 | 6.7 | 6.1 | 6.0 |
| Severe Disab (3-4) | 3.0 | 3.1 | 3.7 | 3.4 | 3.5 |
| Very Severe (5-6) | 3.7 | 3.4 | 3.0 | 3.0 | 2.9 |
| Institutionalized | 6.8 | 6.6 | 6.1 | 5.7 | 4.2 |
| Assisted Living | 0.0 | 0.0 | 0.0 | 0.0 | 2.3 |
| Nursing Home | 6.2 | 5.9 | 5.8 | 5.4 | 3.4 |

NHIS from 1982 to 1996 show strikingly similar declines in disability, again with an accelerated rate of decline in more recent years (Schoeni et al. 2001).

Recently, Freedman and Martin (Freedman et al. 2002) performed a systematic review of 16 studies of trends in disability in the US and found each of them to be consistent in finding declining disability over time. Thus, the literature, although of uneven quality, shows consensus. The NLTCS data had a sample of all Medicare eligibles, both institutionalized and not, covered a sufficient time period (1982-1999), and had well-defined disability measures; this represents the single best study (Fig. 2; Fries 2002).

Multiple causes for this decline in disability appear likely, with no identifiable single cause. Contributions appear probable from reduction in cigarette smoking, medical advances such as better treatment of hypertension, diabetes, coronary artery disease and rheumatoid arthritis, total joint replacements, and medical preventive measures such as colon cancer screening, influenza and pneumococcal vaccines, and cardioprotective-dose aspirin (Cutler 2001). It might be that rising expectations for healthier aging became self-fulfilling, perhaps through a mechanism of perceived self-efficacy (Lorig et al. 2001). There is a strong association of level of education and health, and self-efficacy might be at least part of the explanation for this association; education levels in seniors rose substantially over these past two decades (Bandura 2000). Social factors do not appear to have played a large role in the US; access to care has not improved, and access to prescription drugs may have become more difficult (Cutler 2001). Whatever the reasons, however, compression of morbidity is currently occurring at the population level in the US.

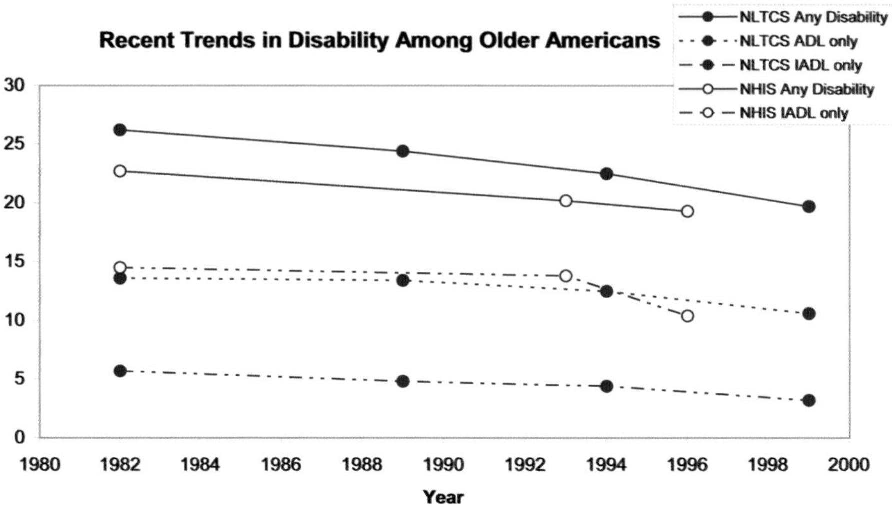


**Fig. 2.** Recent trends in disability among older Americans. Disability rates decline at about 2% per year, with the declines accelerating in the most recent time period in the National Long-Term Care Survey (NLTCS) and the National Health Interview Survey (NHIS). Declines are in both Activities of Daily Living (ADL) and Instrumental Activities of Daily Living (IADL) in the NLTCS. In the NHIS, declines were similar for IADL but not significantly changed for ADL.

## Frailty as the Ultimate Competing Risk for Morbidity and Mortality

Even in this volume, frailty has been defined quite differently by different authors, with different implications. To a physician/biologist, frailty equates with the loss of organ reserve in multiple organs, beginning at or before age 30, at a roughly linear decline of 1.5% per year in the individual organ and an exponential decline in the ability to withstand a perturbation affecting multiple organs. This deline results in a doubling of vulnerability approximately each eight years, known somewhat inaccurately as Gompertz' Law. The frailty phenomenon is perhaps first observed when the champion sprinter or swimmer begins to post slower race times absent injury or reduction in training effort, and it continues through life. In middle life any of us might observe that, despite a regular and focused exercise program and the absence of any apparent disease, our time to run a mile (or performance of some other activity) has drastically increased. When the sporting pages report results of a large marathon by five-year age groups, we observe that the winner in each successive age group was slower than the winner in the immediately younger age group, although we would not conclude that these marathoners had diseases. Or we might observe that our dog is growing older and slower. Or, when visiting a retirement institution for healthy seniors, we note the slow pace of even the most spry 85-year-olds as they walk to lunch. Frailty is physiologic decline, and inevitably it must lead to morbidity, infirmity, and eventually death, as organ reserve is not adequate to withstand even a small perturbation.

Loss of organ reserve can, of course, be accelerated by disease or accident, so the relationship between frailty and medical problems is often not completely obvious. The cigarette smoker accelerates loss of pulmonary organ reserve through disease, the morbidly obese person has accelerated loss of organ reserve in several organs, and paraplegia, Parkinson's disease, and coronary artery disease, among many others, accelerate loss of organ reserve. Some entities often considered diseases, the "degenerative diseases," seem very close to physiologic frailty. Thus, conditions from cataracts to osteoarthritis to benign memory loss do not have causes or cures as the prototypic diseases may, but represent a loss of organ reserve. The frailty we observe clinically is the sum of natural physiologic declines in organ reserve function and disease-related declines in organ reserve, including in this sum those conditions that may be in part disease and in part physiologic decline.

Moreover, physiologic declines, like disease-related declines, can be slowed or even reversed in substantial measure, but not without limit. In general, exercise at a particular activity can improve sub-optimal performance at that activity toward optimal at any age; this conclusion holds for mental, physical, and social activities. Few persons practice or exercise sufficiently to reach their personal limits, and those that do not are capable of improvement. At optimal performance, the principle of the decline of 1.5% per year resumes. These concepts become important especially when considered in the context of the concept of competing risks.

Risks for death and risks for morbidity compete with other risks. This principle is not controversial and is not in dispute, but it is regularly ignored in modeling frailty/morbidity and mortality. Competing risks mandate a dynamic and not a static approach to modeling. People with higher than average levels of risk for one condition tend to have higher than average levels of risk for other conditions. Risks for most conditions, including physiologic frailty, increase exponentially with age. Thus, if you were to remove all risk factors for heart disease, you reduce morbidity and mortality rates, but other risk factors and risks of other diseases rapidly increase over time to take their place. The static approach postulates that if you could remove all diseases and all accidents, an individual or a population could live forever. After considering the dynamic role of competing risks, one can appreciate that the actual effect would be rather dramatically less. Increasing physiologic frailty with age (intrinsic causes) gradually replaces specific diseases (external causes) as a person or a population ages. After acute disease is eliminated, and after chronic disease is eliminated in turn, the limits of the organism are reached. Physiologic frailty is the ultimate competing risk. The limits that it imposes, because of its exponential increases with age, theoretically lead to morbidity compression as reductions in disease incidence permit good health farther into the life span.

## Health Risks and Lifetime Disability

Longitudinal studies of the relationships of lifestyle risk factors to subsequent disability levels in advantaged senior populations are now available. These provide an additional perspective upon the magnitude of postponement of disability that can be expected from population-wide lifestyle changes. Studies of populations with good education levels, relative affluence, and good access to medical care are particularly instructive, since socioeconomic class is otherwise a strong confounding variable. An important issue is whether lifestyle change can provide improvement "at the margin," after medical and social support are already near optimal. Our group is conducting two such ongoing studies: a study of University of Pennsylvania alumni since 1986, when they were enrolled at an average age of 68, and a study of fitness club members and community controls begun in 1984, when participants had an average age of 58.

Effects of good health habits upon subsequent disability were extremely large. In the alumni study, after adjustment for a wide range of possible confounding variables, the cumulative lifetime disability since 1986 was four times as great in those who smoked, were obese, and did not exercise as in lean, exercising nonsmokers. The onset of initial disability was postponed by 7.75 years in the one-third of participants with the best health habits as compared with the worst (Vita et al. 1998). Moreover, in those 418 who had died and whose true total lifetime disability could be computed, those with low health risks had lower disability levels at each year prior to death, albeit with a slow rise over time. Those with higher levels of health risks had more disability throughout the observation period and also showed a rapid surge to higher disability levels in the two years prior to death (Hubert et al. 2002). In the Fitness Club study, using intent-to-treat analyses and after adjustment for co-variates, the initial exercise club cohort had postponement of disability as measured by the Health Assessment Questionnaire (HAQ) of 12.8 years as compared with the more sedentary controls (Wang et al. 2002). The lowest HAQ disability level detectable in an individual is 0.125 on a 0-3 scale; average numbers lower than this thus indicate the presence of a number of individuals with no detectable disability at all (Fig. 3). These postponements of disability far exceed any increases in life expectancy resulting from the better health habits.

## Health Enhancement Interventions

A final metric is examination of the effects of interventions. Is it possible to intervene in senior populations, improve risk factor profiles, and observe improved health and reduced medical care costs? Or would such intervention be "too little, too late?" Large, randomized, controlled trials of health promotion programs in seniors or retirees (Fries et al. 1993, 1994), in particular those that use complex "tailored print interventions" very specific to the participant, have been able to document substantial health improvement. Risk reductions have approximated 10% per year of intervention, and improved self-reported health, decreased disability and pain (Fries et al. 1997), and reduction in medical care utilization, both

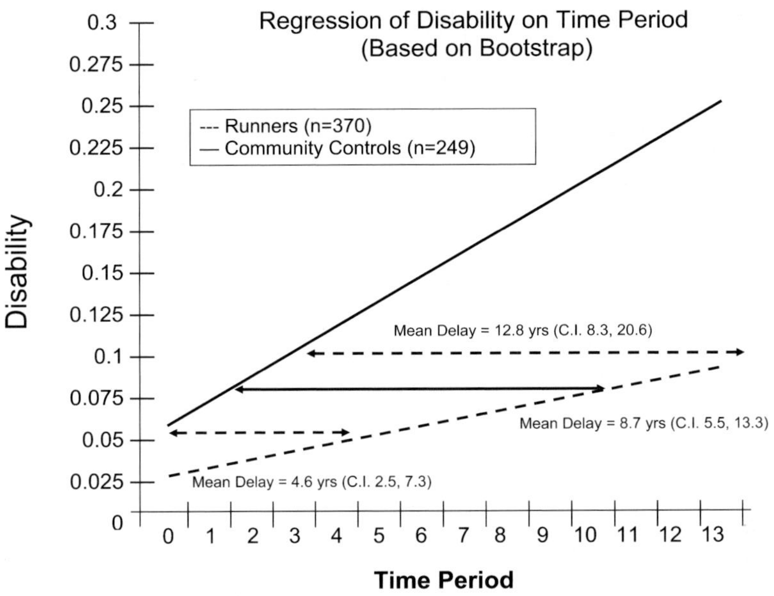


**Fig. 3.** Development of disability over a 13-year period from an average age of 58 in Runner's Club and Community Control groups, with linear regression lines adjusted for co-variates, documenting postponement of disability in the fitness club group compared with controls, with differences increasing over time.

by self-report and analysis of claims, of at least 10% per year have been reported (RAND 2002; Lorig et al. 2001).

## Health Policy Initiatives

Encouragingly, current data on trends in morbidity and mortality suggest that we must be doing something right. The surprise is that this seems to have occurred even though we have not systematically implemented possibly the most promising approach - postponing disability through primary prevention - into health care systems. We now have serial data documenting health improvement over time, and we have monitoring systems in place to observe future trends. We have solid underlying theory from the Compression of Morbidity paradigm, proof of concept by longitudinal epidemiologic studies, and proven interventions that can be broadly applied. While health risk improvement is the most promising single approach to accelerating Compression of Morbidity, it will also be important for us to focus additional efforts on reducing disability from the non-fatal diseases. The most prevalent conditions of later life, such as osteoarthritis, rheumatoid arthritis, depression, isolation, and Alzheimer's disease, have relatively little effect on mortality yet cause an immense amount of morbidity. Progress against disability from these conditions is a particularly leveraged way to accelerate morbidity compression.

Arguably our greatest international national health problem in developed nations is the health of seniors, and one of our greatest economic problems is also the health of seniors. There is an urgent need to find and implement solutions (RAND 2002; Rowe 1999; Fries 2003). In the US, a number of health policy initiatives now target postponement of senior illness and frailty. Healthy Senior bills have been presented in both houses of Congress. This is unprecedented activity and a remarkable opportunity for major change and for major health improvement.

The Compression of Morbidity research agenda includes: 1) more accurate monitoring of disability trends through multi-national survey programs, with addition of more quantitative disability measures and inclusion of quality-of-life measures; 2) more precise definition of the causes behind the trends, possibly using econometric techniques; and3) systematic studies of specific primary prevention interventions, with the goal of identifying those population-based approaches to compression of morbidity that are most effective and most cost-efficient. This agenda, discussed previously (Fries 2003) and elaborated here, has immense implications for the improvement of human health.

## Acknowledgments

This work was supported by grants from the National Institutes of Health to ARAMIS (Arthritis, Rheumatism, and Aging Medical Information System)(AG15815 and AR43584)

## References

Bandura A (2000) Health promotion from the perspective of social cognitive theory. In: Norman P, Abraham C, Conner M. (eds) Understanding and changing health and behaviour.. Harwood, Reading UK pp. 299-339

Bruce B, Fries JF (2003) The Stanford Health Assessment Questionnaire: a review of its history, issues, progress, and documentation. J Rheumatol 30:167-178.

Cutler DM (2001) Declining disability among the elderly. Health Affairs; Nov-Dec: 1-27.

Freedman VA, Martin LG, Schoeni RF (2002) Recent trends in disability and functioning among older adults in the United States: a systematic review. JAMA 288:3137-3146.

Fries JF (1980) Aging, natural death and the compression of morbidity. New Engl J Med 303:130-135.

Fries JF (2002) Reducing disability in older age. JAMA 288:3164-3167.

Fries JF (2003) Measuring and monitoring success in compressing morbidity. Ann Intern Med 39:455-459.

Fries JF, Bloch DA, Harrington H, Richardson N, Beck R (1993). Two-year results of a randomized controlled trial of a health promotion program in a retiree population: the Bank of America study. Am J Med 94:455-462.

Fries JF, Harrington H, Edward R, Kent LA, Richardson N (1994) Randomized controlled trial of cost reductions from a health education program: the California Public Employees Retirement System (CalPERS) study. Am J Health Promotion 8:216-223.

Fries JF, Carey C, McShane DJ (1997) Patient education in arthritis: randomized controlled trial of a mail-delivered program. J Rheumatol 24:1378-1383.

Gruenberg EM (1977) The failure of success. Milbank Mem Fund Q 55:3-24.

Hubert HB, Bloch DA, Oehlert JW, Fries JF (2002) Lifestyle habits and compression of morbidity. J Gerontol 57A:M347-M351.

Kranczer S (1999) Continued United States longevity increases. Statistical Bulletin, Metropolitan Life Oct-Dec:20-27.

Lorig KR, Ritter P, Stewart AL, Sobel DS, Brown BW Jr., Bandura A, Gonzalez VM, Laurent DD, Holman HR (2001) Chronic disease self-management program: 2-year health status and health care utilization outcomes. Med Care 39:1217-1223.

Manton KG, Gu X (2001) Changes in the prevalence of chronic disability in the United States black and non-black population above age 65 from 1982 to 1999. Proc Natl Acad Sci USA 98:6354-6359.

Myers GC, Manton KG (1984). Compression of mortality: myth or reality? Gerontologist 24:346-353.

Olshansky SJ, Ault AB (1986) The fourth stage of the epidemiologic transition: the age of delayed degenerative diseases. Milbank Mem Fund Q 64:355-391.

RAND (2002) Evidence report and evidence-based recommendations: health risk appraisals and Medicare. US Department of Health and Human Services Contract number 500-98-0281. Baltimore, MD 21244-1850

Rowe JW (1999) Geriatrics, prevention, and the remodeling of Medicare. New Engl J Med 340:720-721 (editorial)

Schoeni R, Freedman VA, Wallace R (2001) Persistent, consistent, widespread, and robust? Another look at recent trends in old-age disability. J Gerontol B Psych Sci Soc 56B(supplement): S206-S218.

Singer BH, Manton KG (1998) The effects of health changes on projections of health service needs for the elderly population of the United States. Proc Natl Acad Sci USA 95:15618-15622.

Verbrugge LM (1984) Longer life but worsening health? Trends in health and mortality of middle-aged and older persons. Milbank Mem Fund Q 62:475-519.

Vita AJ, Terry RB, Hubert HB, Fries JF (1998) Aging, health risks, and cumulative disability. New Engl J Med 338:1035-1041.

Wang BWE, Ramey DR, Schettler JD, Hubert HB, Fries JF (2002) Postponed development of disability in senior runners: a 13-year longitudinal study. Arch Int Med 162:2285-2294.

# Cognition and frailty: possible interrelations

*J.-P. Michel*[1,2], *S. Bonin-Guillaume*[1], *G. Gold*[1] *and F. Herrmann*[1]

Over the past century, population aging in developed countries has resulted in a doubling of the population over 60 years. This phenomenon is occurring at an accelerated rate in developing countries, which will undergo a similar demographic change over less than three decades (Kalache 1996). Since 1970, harmonized calculations of "healthy life expectancy" in countries where data are available (Australia, Canada, France, Japan, the United Kingdom and the United States) show that the gains in life expectancy might be several years with any level of disability (Robine et al. 1999). Among the various causes of disability, mental disorders - especially depression in adulthood and dementia in aged adults - are among the leading contributors to "the burden of disease" (Mesle et al. 2000; Vos et al. 2001). In most countries, the prevalence of dementia varies between 6 and 8% among individuals aged 65 years or more and rises dramatically with age. For each decade after the sixth, the number of demented individuals doubles, reaching an estimated rate of 30% of the population aged above 85 (Katchaturian and Radebaugh 1998; Ritchie and Kildea 1995).

Furthermore, in a meta-analysis, Stuck et al. (1999) identified the ten principal risk factors for disability and handicap in community-dwelling old adults. This list included, in alphabetical order, cognitive impairment, co-morbidity, depression, low body mass index, low frequency of social contact, low level of physical activity, lower extremity functional limitation, no alcohol use (vs. moderate), smoking and visual impairment (Stuck et al. 1999).

It has been established that frailty is a significant risk factor for disability (Chin et al. 1999; Guilley et al. 2003) and that both disability and cognitive impairment show similar patterns of increasing frequency with ageing (Barberger-Gateau and Fabrigoule 1997).

Interestingly, health professionals often restrict their conceptualization of frailty to physical domains. Recently, 20 senior geriatricians were asked to list, in order of decreasing importance, 20 subjective items belonging to the "physical frailty domain." Cognitive impairment and depression were considered but were classified in only the eighth and ninth positions (Studenski et al. 2004).

Are physical and functional impairment a possible cause of cognitive decline? Is the reverse also possible? Or are frailty and cognitive decline simply indepen-

[1] Département de Réhabilitation et Gériatrie, Hôpitaux Universitaires de Genève, Université de Genève

[2] Centre Interfacultaire de Gérontologie, Université de Genève, 3, chemin du Pont-Bochet, CH-1226 Thônex-Genève, e-mail: jean-pierre.michel@hcuge.ch

Carey et al.
Longevity and Frailty

dent and coexisting age-related conditions? This paper will address these questions and attempt to clarify the possible interaction between cognition and the onset and development of the frailty process.

## Is physical frailty a risk factor for cognitive decline?

Among other symptoms, non-intentional weight loss is a major identified symptom of physical frailty (Chin et al. 1999; Fried et al. 2001). The 20-year longitudinal study of older community dwelling elders (134 men and 165 women) by Barrett-Connor et al. demonstrated that, compared to those who remained cognitively intact, individuals who developed dementia had a significant non-intentional weight loss after the baseline visit ($P < 0.001$ for men and $P < 0.003$ for women; Barrett-Connor et al. 1996). These data are in concordance with a cross-sectional study of 7,105 community-dwelling 75+-year-old men and women, performed in five different French areas. The goal of this study, called EPIDOS, was to compare the measurement of fat free mass (by dual energy X-ray absorptiometry) with the results of the short, portable mental status questionnaire applied to the same population. Women with the lowest cognitive function had a lower weight ($p < 0.001$), lower fat-free-soft tissue mass ($p = 0.025$), lower fat mass ($p = 0.013$) and lower bone density ($p < 0.001$) compared to women with the highest cognitive function. Another way to express these results is to say that women in the lower quartile of fat-free soft tissue mass had a 43% higher risk of cognitive impairment than those in the highest quartile (Nourhashemi et al. 2002). Furthermore, a body mass index lower than 21 has been described as an early clinical sign of dementia (Nourhashemi et al. 2003). These results suggest that several frailty markers related to nutritional status, such as non-intentional loss of weight, low fat free soft tissue mass and low body mass index (BMI,) are closely associated with the development of cognitive impairment.

Another way to consider the impact of "physical frailty" or, more exactly, the impact of changes in the four Instrumental Activities of Daily Living (IADL) performances (telephone use, use of public transportation, responsibility for medication intake and budget management) on the onset of cognitive decline is to refer to the Paquid study, which consisted of a one-year follow-up of 1,804 non-demented, community-dwelling men and women aged 65+ years. The adjusted odds ratios for the development of dementia over one year, fixed at 1.0 for independent subjects at baseline, increased to 10.6 for dependent subjects in one IADL and 318.4 for those dependent in the four above-mentioned IADLs at inclusion. Thus, impaired IADL, another marker of frailty, was strongly related to dementia incidence in this study (Barberger-Gateau et al. 1993).

## Is cognitive decline a risk factor for physical frailty?

A well-known cross-sectional study of 678 nuns in 1992 and 575 nuns in 1994, comprehensively assessed in both neuropsychological and physical domains, showed that low normal cognitive function at the first assessment doubled the risk of being totally ADL-dependent at the second assessment, in comparison with high cognitive function (Greiner et al. 1996).

The results of a three-year longitudinal survey of 1,856 community-dwelling elderly, free of ADL limitation at baseline and evaluated both by Pfeiffer's Short Portable Mental Status Questionnaire (PSPMSQ) and by changes in ADL performance, showed that, for each error on the PSPMSQ, there was a three-year incidence increase in ADL limitations [O.R. in men = 2.72 (1.36-5.43) and O.R. in women = 2.60 (152-4.44)}, after adjusting for the effects of housing type, age, race, history of chronic health conditions and incident health conditions (Moritz et al. 1995).

These cross-sectional and longitudinal studies strongly suggest that early cognitive decline can lead to impairment in ADL over the ensuing years.

Furthermore, dementing conditions are often associated with affective symptomology that can be present very early in the course of the disease, before the advent of dementia-related functional limitations. In fact, depression may even precede and possibly lead to cognitive changes. In a 12-year follow-up study of 2,812 non-institutionalized elderly with the Centre for Epidemiological Studies Depression Scale and the Short Portable Memory Status Questionnaire (Bassuk et al. 1998), the risk of incident cognitive decline was significantly higher at 3, 6 and 12 years in old adults with symptoms of depression than in those without [three-year O.R = 1.72 (1.04-2.82) vs. 0.93 (0.62-1.00) and six-year O.R, 2.40 (1.33-4.34) vs. 1.03 (0.67-1.58)], after adjustment for age, gender, type of education, income and functional disability (Bassuk et al. 1998).

This finding may be particularly important with regards to the interaction between mild cognitive changes and functional performance, as affective disorders have been shown to decrease functional capacity.

In a WHO one-year longitudinal and collaborative study of 1,051 individuals free of physical disability at baseline, 14% had depressive symptoms at baseline. After controlling for physical disease severity, it appeared that depressive illness resulted in a 1.5-fold (at three months) and a 1.8-fold (at 12 months) increase in the risk of new onset physical disability (Ormel et al. 1999). Similarly, a recent study reported that old subjects with premorbid depressive symptoms who experienced a somatic event had an increased risk of poor adjustment (social and role functioning, well-being, and general health) compared to non depressed elderly (de Jonge et al. 2004).

Depressed mood is also a predictor of decline in physical performance. In a sample of 2,275 non-cognitively impaired men with an average age of 77.1 years participating in the Honolulu Heart Program, Depression (CES_D scale), BMI and maximal hand-grip strength measurements (dynamometer) were assessed at baseline and three years later. After adjusting for baseline strength, age, height, sociodemographic variables and diseases, the odds ratio for steep strength decline was more than four times greater among those who were depressed and underweight, and twice as great among people who were depressed and normal weight, compared with those who were nondepressed and overweight (Rantanen et al. 2000). Furthermore, depressive symptoms may also represent a component of the frailty concept as defined by Fried et al. (2001): exhaustion, low activity (loss of interest), slowness, and weight loss are features of frailty as well as of depression (Katz 2004). This is even more true with atypical geriatric depression such as depression without sadness, depression executive dysfunction syndrome or "subsyndromal depression," characterized by psychomotor retardation, loss of interest, thought slowness and not dysphoric mood (Alexopoulos et al. 2002; Gallo and Rabins 1999; Judd et al. 1994). These late-life depressions are more likely to have poor outcomes in term of relapses and chronicity (Gallo et al. 1997).

## Physical and cognitive decline: a downward spiral?

Are physical and cognitive declines mutually interactive? In a three-year, population-based longitudinal study, 365 community-living adults aged 75+, from different ethnic origins, were screened with the Pfeiffer's Short Portable Mental Status Questionnaire (PSPMSQ) and the ADL performances test. Multivariate regression model analyses were applied to the whole studied sample, to predict the onset of 1) cognitive decline in respondents free of cognitive impairment at baseline, 2) functional decline in respondents free of ADL dependence at baseline, and 3) cognitive and functional declines in respondents with neither at baseline. Several risk factors, such as hypertension, diabetes and low level of education, were identified in all three analyses (Table 1). Importantly, altered cognitive status increased the risk of functional impairment by 50% in group 1, and deficits in ADL in group 2 increased the risk of cognitive deficits. The fact that risk factors were much more strongly related to the combined occurrence of cognitive and functional impairments suggests a synergistic effect (Table 1; Gill et al. 1996).

**Table 1.** Multivariate logistic regression models to predict cognitive, functional, or cognitive and functional decline at a three-year follow-up (N = 289), in respondents free of the specific impairment at baseline.

| | Cognitive decline | | Functional decline | | Cognitive and functional decline | |
|---|---|---|---|---|---|---|
| | OR | IC 95% | OR | IC 95% | OR | IC 95% |
| Female | | | 1.32 | [1.01-1.72] | 2.85 | [1.70-4.79] |
| Age | | | 1.04 | [1.01-1.06] | 1.06 | [1.01-1.11] |
| Education 12 years | | | 2.45 | [1.88-3.19] | 2.43 | [1.26-4.66] |
| Hypertension | 1.67 | [1.34-1.93] | 1.85 | [1.47-2.33] | 6.85 | [4.09-11.46] |
| Diabetes | 1.23 | [1.02-1.42] | 1.69 | [1.18-2.42] | 7.05 | [4.16-11.94] |
| Stroke | 1.26 | [1.04-1.68] | 2.98 | [2.15-4.13] | | |
| Heart disease | | | | | 1.76 | [1.16-2.67] |
| Hip fracture | 1.85 | [1.30-2.63] | | | | |
| ADL disability | 1.57 | [1.26-1.95] | | | 1.19 | [1.09-1.31] |
| SPMSQ errors | | | 1.09 | [1.03-1.15] | 1.08 | [1.02-1.50] |

Cognitive and functional impairments thus appear complimentary, each precipitating the decline of the other.

## Conclusions

The frailty concept should not be limited to physical domains. As recently pointed out, "the consensus around physical frailty has to begin by identifying its own content" (Studenski et al. 2004). We are convinced that the frailty concept includes several interconnected domains, such as mobility, energy, sensory abilities, physical symptoms and also mental disturbances, including anxiety, depression, and cognitive impairment, which are very frequent in the extreme age of life. In this global context, frailty should be viewed as a dynamic process and its interactions with cognition and depression should be taken into consideration. Further studies in the field should address these issues.

## References


Alexopoulos GS, Meyers BS, Young RC, Kalayam B, Kakuma T, Gabrielle M, Sirey JA, Hull J (2000) Executive dysfunction and long-term outcomes of geriatric depression. Arch Gen Psychiatry 57: 285-290

Alexopoulos GS, Kiosses DN, Klimstra S, Kalayam B, Bruce ML (2002) Clinical presentation of the "depression-executive dysfunction syndrome" of late life. Am J Geriatr Psychiat 10: 98-106.

Barberger-Gateau P, Fabrigoule C (1997) Disability and cognitive impairment in the elderly. Disabil Rehabil 19: 175-193

Barberger-Gateau P, Dartigues JF, Letenneur L (1993) Four Instrumental Activities of Daily Living Score as a predictor of one-year incident dementia. Age Ageing 22, 457-463.

Barrett-Connor E, Edelstein SL, Corey-Bloom J, Wiederholt WC (1996) Weight loss precedes dementia in community-dwelling older adults. J Am Geriatr Soc, 44: 1147-1152.

Bassuk SS, Berkman LF, Wypij D (1998) Depressive symptomatology and incident cognitive decline in an elderly community sample. Arch Gen Psychiat 55: 1073-1081.

Chin A, Paw MJ., Dekker JM, Feskens EJ, Schouten EG, Kromhout D (1999) How to select a frail elderly population? A comparison of three working definitions. J Clin Epidemiol 52: 1015-1021.

de Jonge P, Ormel J, Slaets JP, Kempen GI, Ranchor AV, van Jaarsveld CH, Scaf-Klomp W, Sanderman R. (2004) Depressive symptoms in elderly patients predict poor adjustment after somatic events. Am J Geriatr Psychiat 12: 57-64.

Fried L.P, Tangen CM, Walston J, Newman AB, Hirsch C, Gottdiener J, Seeman T, Tracy R, Kop WJ, Burke G, McBurnie MA (2001) Frailty in older adults: evidence for a phenotype. J Gerontol A Biol Sci Med Sci 56: M146-156.

Gallo JJ, Rabins PV (1999) Depression without sadness: alternative presentations of depression in late life. Am Fam Physician 60: 820-826.

Gallo JJ, Rabins PV, Lyketsos CG, Tien AY., Anthony JC (1997). Depression without sadness: functional outcomes of nondysphoric depression in later life. J Am Geriatr Soc 45: 570-578.

Gill TM, Williams CS, Richardson ED, Tinetti ME (1996) Impairments in physical performance and cognitive status as predisposing factors for functional dependence among nondisabled older persons. J Gerontol A Biol Sci Med Sci 51: M283-288.

Greiner PA, Snowdon DA, Schmitt FA (1996). The loss of independence in activities of daily living: the role of low normal cognitive function in elderly nuns. Am J Publ Health 86: 62-66.

Guilley E, Armi F, Ghisletta P, Lalive d'Epinay C, Michel J (2003) Vers une définition opérationnelle de la fragilité. Méd Hyg 61: 2256-2261.

Judd LL, Rapaport MH, Paulus MP, Brown JL (1994) Subsyndromal symptomatic depression: a new mood disorder? J Clin Psychiat 55 (Suppl): 18-28.

Kalache A (1996) Ageing world-wide. In: B.M.S.P. Group (edd) Epidemiology in old age. London, pp. 22-31.

Katchaturian ZS, Radebaugh TS (1998) AD: Where are we now? Where are we going? Alzheimer Dis Ass Disord 1998: 12; Suppl 3 S24–8.

we going? Alzheimer Dis Assoc Disord 12(suppl 3): S24–S28.

Katz IR (2004) Depression and frailty: the need for multidisciplinary research. Am J Geriatr Psychiat 12(1): 1-6.

Melse JM, Essink-Bot ML, Kramers PG, Hoeymans N (2000) A national burden of disease calculation: Dutch disability-adjusted life-years. Dutch Burden of Disease Group. Am J Publ Health 90: 1241-1247.

Moritz DJ, Kasl SV, Berkman LF (1995) Cognitive functioning and the incidence of limitations in activities of daily living in an elderly community sample. Am J Epidemiol 141: 41-49.

Nourhashemi F, Andrieu S, Gillette-Guyonnet S, Reynish E, Albarede JL, Grandjean H, Vellas B (2002) Is there a relationship between fat-free soft tissue mass and low cognitive function? Results from a study of 7,105 women. J Am Geriatr Soc 50: 1796-1801.

Nourhashemi F, Deschamps V, Larrieu S, Letenneur L., Dartigues JF, Barberger-Gateau P (2003) Body mass index and incidence of dementia: the PAQUID study. Neurology 60: 117-119.

Ormel J, Vonkorff M, Oldehinkel AJ., Simon G, Tiemens BG, Ustun TB (1999) Onset of disability in depressed and non-depressed primary care patients. Psychol Med 29: 847-853.

Rantanen T, Penninx BW, Masaki K, Lintunen T, Foley D, Guralnik JM (2000). Depressed mood and body mass index as predictors of muscle strength decline in old men. J Am Geriatr Soc 48: 613-617.

Ritchie K, Kildea D (1995) Is senile dementia "age-related" or "aging related"? Evidence from meta-analysis of dementia prevalence in the oldest old. Lancet 1995; 346: 931-934.

Robine JM, Romieu I, Cambois E (1999) Health expectancy indicators. Bull World Health Org 77: 181-185.

Stuck AE, Walthert JM, Nikolaus T, Bula CJ, Hohmann C, Beck JC (1999) Risk factors for functional status decline in community-living elderly people: a systematic literature review. Soc Sci Med 1999; 48: 445-469.

Studenski S, Hayes RP, Leibowitz RQ, Bode R, Lavery L, Walston J, Duncan P, Pererra S (2004) Clinical global impression of change in physical frailty: development of a measure based on clinical judgment. J Am Geriatr Assoc 2004; 52: 1560-1566.

Vos T, Mathers C, Herrman H, Harvey C, Gureje O, Bui D, Watson N, Begg S (2001) The burden of mental disorders in Victoria, 1996. Soc Psychiatry Psychiatr Epidemiol 36: 53-62.

# Consequences of the 2003 summer heat wave on mortality levels in France

*E. Jougla*[1] *and D. Hémon*[2]

## Introduction

For the first two weeks of August 2003, France sweltered under a heat wave of exceptional duration and intensity (Hemon and Jougla 2003; Météo-France 2003). Only days after it began, information from various sources – hospital emergency rooms, fire departments, paramedical emergency services, and funeral homes – showed a brutal rise in mortality and in recourse to emergency services (InVS 2003). On August 20, the Minister of Health appointed a committee to assess the scale and epidemiologic characteristics of the excess mortality associated with the heat wave, to study the factors of vulnerability to exposure to heat waves, and to propose changes in the alert system.

This article summarizes the principal results of this committee's first progress report and responds to the following questions:

- what was the chronological development and extent of the excess mortality in August 2003?
- what was the relation between mortality and temperature characteristics ?
- how was the excess mortality distributed according to sex, age, geography and site of death?
- what causes of death were most common?

## Material and methods

### General approach

Several epidemiologic studies have already described the short-term excess mortality that has accompanied heat waves in different countries (Besancenot 2002; Basu and Samet 2002). They show that the excess mortality is not limited to deaths that are directly linked to exposure to excessive heat, dehydration, hyperthermia, or heatstroke, but also involves a wide variety of causes of death. To estimate the excess mortality, therefore, we compared the deaths during August 2003 with

[1] INSERM-CépiDc – IFR 69 – Centre d'Epidémiologie sur les causes médicales de décès, Le Vésinet, France

[2] INSERM-U170 – IFR 69 – Recherches épidémiologiques et statistiques sur l'environnement et la santé, Villejuif, Franc

Carey et al.
Longevity and Frailty

corresponding data from the previous three summers. In view of the information collected, the analysis specifically covered mortality from August 1–28 and characterized in more detail the mortality from August 1–20, the days with more deaths than expected.

## Data sources and counting deaths

Strict monitoring of the exhaustiveness of the death counts required combining information from different sources: death certificates and vital status "7" bulletins (source: INSERM), vital status "7-bis" notices (source: INSEE), and death counts from the district health departments (DDASS; source: InVS). A death certificate stating the cause of death is transmitted to the municipal vital statistics office by the physician who certifies the death. The "7" bulletin is completed by the same office when the death is reported. The certificate is anonymous (that is, it omits the decedent's name), but it does include his or her social and demographic characteristics: sex, date of birth and death, and place of death. The municipality sends both the death certificate and the "7" bulletin to the DDASS, which transmits them to INSERM. It also transmits the "7-bis" notice, which includes the subject's name but is otherwise identical to the "7" bulletin, to INSEE. The transmission of all these documents was accelerated at the beginning of the third week of August, and the DDASS transmitted their death counts daily to InVS by email in August. The death counts for the period of August 1–31 furnished by the combination of INSERM and INSEE sources (56,387 deaths) and by InVS (56,146 death) are extremely close (Table 1). Together these three sources provide an exhaustive list of the deaths occurring between August 1 and 28.

## Reference values for mortality

The number of deaths observed in August 2003 was compared with reference values, which were estimated according to three methods:

- the mean number of daily deaths observed in July, August and September in 2000, 2001, and 2002;
- the number of deaths obtained by applying the July–September mortality rate for 2000–2002 to population estimates as of June 30, 2003;
- the number of deaths expected by applying the mortality rate from a model of trends in mortality over the past ten years (1993–2002) for metropolitan France, by age and sex, to population estimates as of June 30, 2003.

To assess the validity of these methods, we estimated the number of deaths expected in the months of April and May 2003 with all three methods and compared them with the number of deaths actually observed. The first method estimated the number of expected deaths most exactly and was applied to the analysis. Moreover, it is not based on population estimates or on any modeling of mortality rate trends and it allows us to conduct the planned statistical analyses of epidemiologic characteristics.

**Table 1.** Number of deaths recorded by the three information sources: InVs, INSEE, INSERM

| | InVs | INSEE | | | INSERM | INSERM / INSEE |
|---|---|---|---|---|---|---|
| | | Computer-equipped municipalities (CM) | | 7 bis | | |
| | Sept 17 | 781 CM Sept 17 (a) | Estimate for France nationwide ( a / 0.646) | 7 bis Sept 12 | "7 CépiDC" Sept 17 | "7 CépiDc / 7 Bis" Sept 17 |
| August 1-31 | 56,146 | 36,121.0 | 55,914.86 | 54,542 | 55,340 | 56,387 |
| August 1-20 | 41,568 | 26,766.0 | 41,433.44 | 40,583 | 40,923 | 41,621 |
| August 21-28 | 10,836 | 6,951.0 | 10,760.06 | 10,453 | 10,759 | 10,957 |
| August 1-28 | 52,404 | 3,3717 | 52,193.50 | 51,036 | 51,682 | 52,578 |

## Indicators and variables

Two indicators were used to characterize mortality: the mortality ratio (O/E = number of deaths observed relative to the number expected) and excess mortality (O - E = the difference between the number of observed and expected deaths). Given the negligible variations in the population between 2000 and 2003, the mortality ratio measures the ratio of the mortality rate observed in August 2003 to that during the reference period (2000–2002). The excess mortality measures the absolute difference between the number of deaths observed in August 2003 and the number expected according to the reference mortality in 2000–2002. These indicators were analyzed according to sex, age, region, district and site (home, hospital, private clinic, retirement or nursing home, public place) of death. The study of causes of death was based on the analysis of all coded death certificates. These medical data are compared with those from 2000 and 2001, the most recent years for which a validated analysis of causes of death is available. Daily maximum and minimum temperatures, both nationwide and by district, come from Météo-France and were recorded at 180 Météo-France weather stations situated throughout the country and representative of the climate.

# Results

## Characteristics of the heat wave

For the first half of August 2003 (Hemon and Jougla 2003), France sweltered under a heat wave that was exceptional in its duration (nearly two weeks) and intensity. For each of the first 12 days, the maximum temperature every day broke records dating back to the 19th century and to the earliest records. Starting on August 4, two thirds of the 180 Météo-France weather stations reported temperatures exceeding 35°C. Temperatures exceeded 35° for an exceptional number of days in an exceptional geographic range. Temperatures above 40°C were observed in 15% of the weather stations, including in Brittany. More than 80 districts endured a temperature above 35° for at least one day and 61 districts for at least nine days. The chronology of mean maximum temperatures for all the Météo-France weather stations shows that the maximum temperatures rose progressively from August 1 to 5 from a value near the norm (25°C) to a value of 37°C, remained between 36°C and 37°C through August 13, and then regressed rapidly in the days that followed (28°C on August 16).

## Chronology and estimated excess mortality

In most of the country, the wave of excess mortality began on August 4. On that day alone, there were nearly 300 more deaths than in the previous years, although the normal margin of variation of the daily number of deaths in summer months is approximately 150 deaths. The daily excess increased regularly and massively, reaching 1,200 deaths on August 8 and nearly 2,200 on August 12 (Fig. 1). It began to regress on August 13; there were roughly 2,000 deaths in excess on the August 13 and 1,000 the next day. Mortality levels progressively declined, returning to their normal value on August 19. The cumulative number of excess deaths from the beginning of August was 400 on August 4, 3,900 on August 8, 10,600 on August 12, and 14,800 on August 20 (Fig. 2). The period of excess mortality thus matched the period of the heat wave that scorched France from August 4–13. Excess mortality began to fall after the temperature did and stabilized around August 20, at a cumulative excess mortality of almost 15,000 deaths.

## Excess mortality by sex and age

Globally, mortality from August 1–20 was more than 60% higher than expected (Table 2). It was highest among those aged 75 years or older (+70%) but evident also among those aged 45–74 years (+30%). It remains difficult to determine if mortality increased significantly among those younger than 45 years, since the estimates are more uncertain for lower ages. The mortality ratio was 15–20% higher among women than men in all age groups. Because of this gap and women's generally greater longevity, excess mortality was more than 80% higher among women (+ 9,510 deaths) than men (+ 5,292 deaths).

## Geographic disparities

The excess mortality from August 1–20 affected almost the entire country, but its intensity varied markedly between regions, with mortality ratios ranging from 1.2 to 2.3. Mortality increased by more than 80% across a vast territory,

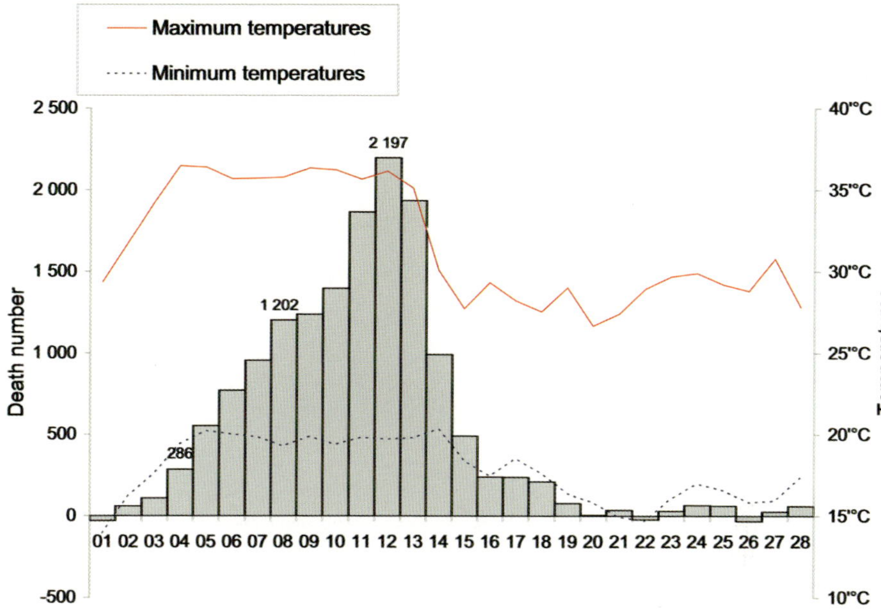


**Fig. 1.** Excess deaths observed daily in August 2003 and exterior temperatures

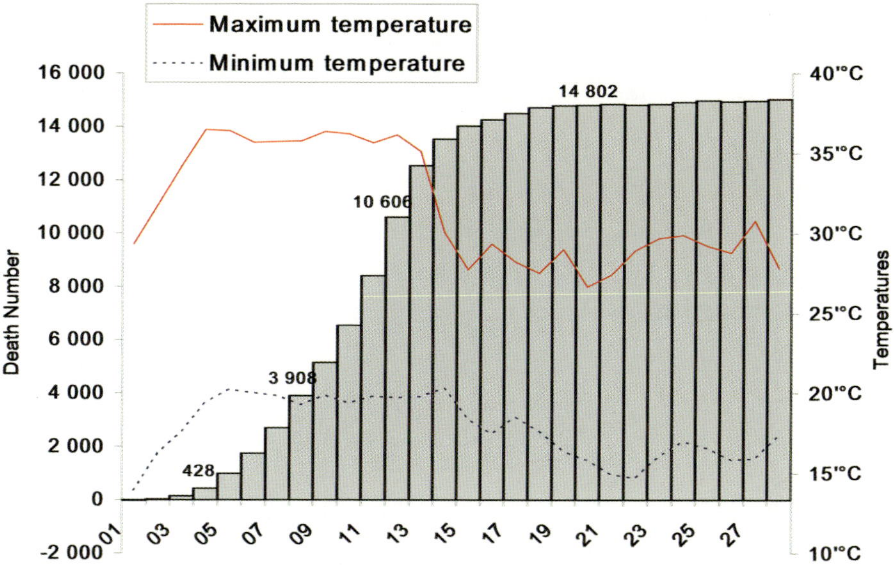


**Fig. 2.** Cumulative excess deaths in August 2003 and exterior temperatures

**Table 2.** Distribution of deaths by age and sex from August 1–20, 2003

| | Women | | | | Men | | | | Total | | | |
|---|---|---|---|---|---|---|---|---|---|---|---|---|
| | O | E | O/E | O-E | O | E | O/E | O-E | O | E | O/E | O-E |
| < 44 years | 538 | 547 | 1.0 | –9 | 1,310 | 1,159 | 1.1 | 151 | 1,848 | 1,706 | 1.1 | 142 |
| < 1 year | 72 | 76 | 0.9 | | 105 | 95 | 1.1 | | 177 | 171 | 1.0 | |
| 1–14 years | 45 | 41 | 1.1 | | 59 | 58 | 1.0 | | 104 | 99 | 1.0 | |
| 15–24 years | 60 | 66 | 0.9 | | 208 | 191 | 1.1 | | 268 | 257 | 1.0 | |
| 25–34 years | 91 | 101 | 0.9 | | 275 | 270 | 1.0 | | 366 | 371 | 1.0 | |
| 35–44 years | 270 | 262 | 1.0 | | 663 | 545 | 1.2 | | 933 | 807 | 1.2 | |
| 45–74 years | 3,896 | 2,852 | 1.4 | 1,044 | 7,345 | 5,939 | 1.2 | 1,406 | 11,241 | 8,791 | 1.3 | 2,450 |
| 45–54 years | 646 | 543 | 1.2 | | 1,566 | 1,255 | 1.2 | | 2,212 | 1,798 | 1.2 | |
| 55–64 years | 995 | 695 | 1.4 | | 2,070 | 1,633 | 1.3 | | 3,065 | 2,328 | 1.3 | |
| 65–74 years | 2,255 | 1,614 | 1.4 | | 3,709 | 3,050 | 1.2 | | 5,964 | 4,664 | 1.3 | |
| ≥ 75 years | 18,018 | 9,543 | 1.9 | 8,475 | 10,514 | 6,779 | 1.6 | 3,735 | 28,532 | 16,322 | 1.7 | 12,210 |
| 75–84 years | 6,414 | 3,417 | 1.9 | | 6,169 | 3,919 | 1.6 | | 12,583 | 7,336 | 1.7 | |
| 85–94 years | 8,878 | 4,924 | 1.8 | | 3,748 | 2,564 | 1.5 | | 12,626 | 7,488 | 1.7 | |
| ≥ 95 years | 2,726 | 1,202 | 2.3 | | 597 | 296 | 2.0 | | 3,323 | 1,498 | 2.2 | |
| Total | 22,452 | 12,942 | 1.7 | 9,510 | 19,169 | 13,877 | 1.4 | 5,292 | 41,621 | 26,819 | 1.6 | 14,802 |

including all the districts of Ile-de-France and a part of the regions of Centre, Champagne-Ardenne, Burgundy, the Loire Valley, and Poitou-Charentes (Table 3). Excess mortality was highest – more than doubled – in Ile-de-France and in Centre. Ile-de-France alone contributed 33% of the national excess deaths; they were high throughout the region, but worst in the districts of Essonne, Hauts-de-Seine, Seine-Saint-Denis, and Val de Marne (excess mortality greater than 150%). The lowest mortality ratios were observed in the coastal regions of Lower-Normandy, Brittany and Nord-Pas de Calais. The rate of excess deaths was also less marked than the national mean in regions where summers are habitually very hot – Languedoc-Roussillon, PACA, Corsica, and Midi-Pyrénées. Excess mortality affected those aged 45-74 years as well as those 75 years or older in all regions. It was nonetheless especially impressive among people 75 or older in the area of the maximum excess mortality, ranging from +142% to +245% according to district.

**Table 3.** Regional distribution of deaths from August 1-20, 2003

| Regions | Number of deaths observed (O) | Number of deaths expected (E) | Excess: O - E | Contribution to global excess (%) | O/E |
|---|---|---|---|---|---|
| Metropolitan France | 41,621 | 26,818.6 | 14,802.4 | 100.0 | 1.6 |
| Alsace | 1,023 | 748.0 | 275.0 | 1.9 | 1.4 |
| Aquitaine | 2,191 | 1,567.0 | 624.0 | 4.2 | 1.4 |
| Auvergne | 1,022 | 747.4 | 274.6 | 1.9 | 1.4 |
| Lower Normandy | 822 | 697.2 | 124.8 | 0.8 | 1.2 |
| Burgundy | 1,477 | 885.1 | 591.9 | 4.0 | 1.7 |
| Brittany | 1,855 | 1,549.9 | 305.1 | 2.1 | 1.2 |
| Centre | 2,441 | 1,203.4 | 1,237.6 | 8.4 | 2.0 |
| Champagne-Ardenne | 988 | 629.1 | 358.9 | 2.4 | 1.6 |
| Corsica | 191 | 143.4 | 47.6 | 0.3 | 1.3 |
| Franche-Comté | 687 | 494.7 | 192.3 | 1.3 | 1.4 |
| Haute-Normandy | 1,066 | 764.3 | 301.7 | 2.0 | 1.4 |
| Ile-de-France | 8,506 | 3,639.1 | 4,866.9 | 32.9 | 2.3 |
| Languedoc-Roussillon | 1,536 | 1,265.9 | 270.1 | 1.8 | 1.2 |
| Limousin | 651 | 469.9 | 181.1 | 1.2 | 1.4 |
| Lorraine | 1,526 | 1,066.4 | 459.6 | 3.1 | 1.4 |
| Midi-Pyrénées | 1,762 | 1,324.5 | 437.5 | 3.0 | 1.3 |
| Nord-Pas-de-Calais | 2,175 | 1,792.3 | 382.7 | 2.6 | 1.2 |
| Pays de Loire | 2,399 | 1,430.9 | 968.1 | 6.5 | 1.7 |
| Picardy | 1,153 | 817.9 | 335.1 | 2.3 | 1.4 |
| Poitou Charente | 1,432 | 872.0 | 560.0 | 3.8 | 1.6 |
| PACA | 3,194 | 2,375.1 | 818.9 | 5.5 | 1.3 |
| Rhône-Alpes | 3,524 | 2,335.3 | 1,188.7 | 8.0 | 1.5 |

## Temporal and spatial relations between exposure to heat and excess mortality

Daily indicators of excess mortality and temperature in the 22 regions were graphed together. In the regions with the highest excess mortality, the daily high and low temperatures increased abruptly in the first days of August, remained high throughout the heat wave and began to fall on August 13. This was the case in Ile-de-France, Centre and Burgundy. Temperatures were high for the entire month of August in the south, but excess mortality remained moderate there. This was the case in the regions of Corsica, Languedoc-Roussillon and Provence-Alpes-Côte d'Azur. In some regions, especially Haute-Normandy and Picardy, but also, although to a lesser extent, in Nord-Pas de Calais, Lower Normandy and Brittany, the heat wave appeared in two phases, separated by a partial and temporary regression of temperatures on August 7 and 8. In these regions, excess mortality also presented very strikingly, two phases that were synchronized with the temperature trends.

The excess mortality observed in the continental districts is clearly associated with the number of days of very hot weather (high temperature at least 35°C and daily low temperature at least 20°C) observed between August 1 and 20: +30% in the districts with zero or one day of very hot weather, +50% for two to five days and +80% for six days or more.

## Site of death

The highest mortality ratios were observed in retirement homes (number of deaths doubled, to 2,640 more deaths than expected) and at home (seven-fold increase, 4,857 excess deaths; Table 4). Next came hospitals (1.5-fold increase, 5,866 excess deaths) and private clinics (two-fold increase, 461 excess deaths). The number of deaths in public places did not change from earlier years. This ranking according to site of death was the same for both sexes and all age groups. The largest increases were seen among women older than 75 years who died in retirement homes or their own homes (the latter more than doubled). Regardless of the place of death, mortality increased more among women and among those 75 years or older. In all (Table 5), 42% of the excess deaths occurred in hospitals, 35% at home, 19% in retirement homes or hospices and 3% in private clinics (compared with, respectively, 53%, 28%, 10% and 9% of deaths in the preceding years). This distribution is similar for men and women. We note nonetheless that women died more often than men in retirement homes (22% vs 13%) as did those 75 years or older (24% instead of 15% for those younger than 75 years). These results must be interpreted with prudence, to the extent that many factors, especially health status, play a role in determining the specific premises where death occurs.

**Table 4.** Excess mortality observed from August 1-20, 2003 in France according to site of death

| | All ages | | | < 75 years | | | ≥ 75 years | | |
|---|---|---|---|---|---|---|---|---|---|
| Site of death | Total | Men | Women | Total | Men | Women | Total | Men | Women |
| Home | 1.7 | 1.5 | 1.9 | 1.4 | 1.4 | 1.6 | 1.9 | 1.6 | 2.1 |
| Hospitals | 1.5 | 1.3 | 1.6 | 1.2 | 1.2 | 1.2 | 1.6 | 1.5 | 1.7 |
| Private clinics | 1.2 | 1.2 | 1.3 | 1.0 | 1.0 | 1.1 | 1.3 | 1.3 | 1.4 |
| Retirement home | 2.0 | 1.8 | 2.1 | 1.8 | 1.8 | 1.9 | 2.0 | 1.8 | 2.1 |
| Public place | 1.0 | 1.0 | 0.9 | 1.0 | 1.0 | 0.9 | 1.0 | 0.9 | 1.1 |

Ratio of deaths from August 1-20, 2003 to mean deaths from 2000-2002 (e.g., 1.7 signifies that the number of deaths at home was 1.7 times larger than in the three previous years for all ages)

**Table 5.** Distribution of excess deaths from August 1-20, 2003 (%) according to site of death – all ages

| | Total | | Men | | Women | |
|---|---|---|---|---|---|---|
| Site of death | Number of excess deaths | % | Number of excess deaths | % | Number of excess deaths | % |
| Home | 4,857 | 35 | 1,809 | 37 | 3,04834 | 34 |
| Hospitals | 5,866 | 42 | 2,280 | 46 | 3,586 | 40 |
| Private clinics | 461 | 3 | 187 | 4 | 274 | 3 |
| Retirement home | 2,640 | 19 | 638 | 13 | 2,002 | 22 |
| All | 13,824 | 100 | 4,914 | 100 | 8,910 | 100 |

The deaths whose site is not reported are not included in this table (35 means that 35% of the excess deaths among men occurred at home)

## Causes of death

We analyzed the causes of all the deaths that occurred in metropolitan France between August 1 and 20 (41,621 death certificates). Mortality ratios (O/E) were highest for causes of death directly attributable to heat (heatstroke, dehydration, hyperthermia). There were 3,468 deaths from these causes observed in 2003 and only 163 deaths during the same period in 2000–2001. Accordingly, the mortality ratio rose substantially (number of deaths multiplied by 20). These causes of death were followed by diseases of the nervous, genitourinary, respiratory, and circulatory systems. Most other causes of death also occurred in greater than expected numbers, but with increases that were less marked for tumors, suicides and other violent deaths. Excess mortality was greater among women for most causes. The women's higher age does not completely explain this trend, since we still find this excess of deaths among women when we limit the analysis to those 75 years or older. Mortality ratios for all diseases were higher in subjects aged 75 years or more than among younger subjects. Overall (Table 6), diseases directly associated with the heat wave – hyperthermia, heatstroke, and dehydration – account for 23% of the excess deaths, diseases of the circulatory system for 21%, diseases of the respiratory system for 9% and cancer for 6%. The analysis of causes of deaths

**Table 6.** Contribution of specific causes of death (%) to general excess mortality (death observed from August 1-20, 2003

| Causes of death | Causes of excess deaths in 2003 | | | Causes of death in 2000–2001 | | |
|---|---|---|---|---|---|---|
| | Total % | Men % | Women % | Total % | Men % | Women % |
| Heat stroke, dehydration, hyperthermia... | 23 | 19 | 25 | 1 | 0 | 1 |
| Diseases of the circulatory system | 21 | 19 | 22 | 29 | 26 | 32 |
| Respiratory system diseases | 9 | 12 | 8 | 5 | 6 | 5 |
| Tumors | 6 | 8 | 6 | 30 | 35 | 25 |
| Mental Illness | 5 | 6 | 5 | 3 | 3 | 4 |
| Diseases of the nervous system | 7 | 7 | 7 | 4 | 3 | 4 |
| Diabetes | 3 | 3 | 3 | 2 | 2 | 2 |
| Infectious diseases | 3 | 3 | 4 | 2 | 2 | 2 |
| Violent deaths (accidents, suicide, homicide) | 3 | 3 | 3 | 8 | 10 | 7 |
| Diseases of the genitourinary system | 3 | 2 | 3 | 2 | 1 | 2 |
| Diseases of the gastrointestinal system | 2 | 3 | 2 | 5 | 5 | 5 |
| Other | 15 | 15 | 12 | 10.2 | 7.5 | 12.9 |
| All | 100 | 100 | 100 | 100.0 | 100.0 | 100.0 |

Percentage of the number of deaths observed from August 1-20, 2003 compared with the total number of deaths observed.(The percentage of 21 calculated for diseases of the circulatory system (total) means that these diseases are responsible for 21% of the excess mortality in 2003. In 2000-2001, diseases of the circulatory system were responsible for 29% of the deaths during the same period.)

associated with the heat wave thus demonstrates clearly a profound modification of the ranking of causes of death that are usually observed (in the previous years, cancers accounted for one third of the deaths).

## Discussion

The preceding analyses make several facts quite clear. In the first two weeks of August 2003, France experienced a heat wave of unprecedented intensity and duration, accompanied by an equally unprecedented wave of excess short-term mortality. These deaths principally struck the elderly populations, especially those 75 years or older but also those aged 45–74 years. They affected men and women, but especially women. The excess deaths were distributed unequally across the country, with the Centre and Ile-de-France regions struck hardest. The districts exposed longest to the heat showed the most marked excess mortality. Deaths at home and in retirement homes doubled. The causes of death that increased most are directly attributable to the heat: dehydration, hyperthermia, and heatstroke.

Some of these results require more detailed analysis. In particular, explaining the excess mortality among women versus men necessitates the study of the factors of "isolation," by relating it to matrimonial status, place of death and cause of death. The effect of the heat wave among younger populations was difficult to assess in this initial study because of the small number of subjects. Further study is needed. The municipality of the decedent's domicile, as well as that where death occurred, will also need to be taken into account. To characterize exactly the health status of the populations most affected (prevalence of serious co-morbidities), we must complete the analysis of all the causes mentioned on death certificates and not only of the single underlying cause.

Météo-France stresses the importance of the heat waves in 1976 and 1983 among those documented in France over the past half century. Unlike the 1983 heat wave, concentrated in the Bouches-du-Rhône, the 1976 heat wave, like the one in 2003, affected a large swath of the country: the Southwest, West, Ile-de-France and Champagne. The hot peak lasted approximately 10 days, from late June through early July. The study of summer deaths since the 1970s shows a clear and unusual excess mortality of very strong amplitude between the last week of June and the first week of July 1976. Although it does not reach the level of 2003, the excess mortality (compared with the mean of 1973–1975) is quite marked, with a total of 6,000 extra deaths (+30%). The day-to-day mortality profile is similar to that observed in 2003. The same populations were struck hardest: the elderly and women (especially very old women). Young children were not affected, but excess death affected all of those 15 years or older. The number of excess deaths was distributed as follows: hospital (43%), home (33%), retirement homes (13%), private clinics (4%) and other (17%). Comparing these figures with those for 2003, we note especially the lower rate of deaths at home. Excess mortality was highest in Paris and the Paris metropolitan area and affected two categories of causes of death most: respiratory diseases and cerebrovascular accidents. Tumor deaths increased little if at all. The especially strong impact of deaths from cerebrovascular accidents was not observed in the 2003 analysis.

A brutal short-term rise in mortality with the onset of heat waves has also been observed in other countries (Basu and Samet 2002; Ellis et al. 1975; MMWR 1994; Katsouyanni et al. 1988; Oechsli and Buechley 1970; Rooney et al. 1998; Sartor et al. 1995; Smoyer 1998; Whitman et al. 1997). Epidemiologic analyses show the importance of the intensity and duration of heat waves and the increase in excess mortality with age, especially with sex (in the European studies), and in large metropolitan urban areas. Nonetheless, none were as exceptional in their duration, intensity and geographic range as the August 2003 heat wave in France. Similarly, the number of excess deaths is not of the same order. The causes of death that rose most often during these heat waves were cerebrovascular, ischemic heart, and respiratory diseases.

Overall, although a crude increase in short-term mortality has long been associated with heat waves, this analysis reveals the exceptional scale of the August 2003 heat wave in France – in its duration and its geographic range, the amplitude of the excess mortality that accompanied it and the constancy of the principal epidemiologic characteristics of excess mortality associated with it.

## Conclusion and perspectives

### Additional work

This initial and purely descriptive analysis of short-term excess mortality associated with the August 2003 heat wave will be completed by more detailed analyses. Their objectives will include:

- simultaneous consideration of the different elements considered separately at this stage descriptive (age, sex, temperatures, cause of death, premises of death ...),
- specification of the quantitative relations between temperature and increase in mortality as a function of population characteristics and environment.

The study will also examine the level and characteristics of mortality through the end of 2003. The potential long-term effects of the heat wave may have taken two opposite forms. Mortality may have increased during the months following this episode if ill or very elderly people who did not die during the peak of the heat wave were weakened by it. Inversely, the heat wave may have accelerated, or displaced, the deaths of those already in very poor health, and reduced mortality levels may therefore be observed in the following months. It will nonetheless not be simple to identify these two potential factors solely on the basis of analysis of the longer-term trends and characteristics of mortality. It will require a simultaneous, very detailed study of the causes of death and specific surveys (based on the medical files of the people who died).

Finally, the relation between mortality and temperature over the past 35 years will be studied in more detail to quantify it and obtain information essential to the implementation of an early health alert system based on analysis of daily climate trends.

## Analysis of other determinants of excess mortality

Epidemiologic analyses of the consequences of past heat waves elsewhere have clearly demonstrated the essential role of the heat wave's intensity and duration but they have also shown the importance of factors such as social characteristics and extent of isolation. Specific aspects of housing are also described as important factors in excess mortality: poor ventilation, lack of air conditioning, building density, urban heat islands. These studies also demonstrate the impact of excessive drug consumption, especially tranquilizers. Air quality, pollution, humidity and heat all act in synergy with rising temperatures. High daily minimum temperatures play an important role by preventing nocturnal recovery. Similarly, the normal temperatures to which the population is accustomed play an important role in their vulnerability to heat waves. The respective role of each of these factors must be studied in specific surveys.

## Alert procedures

The mortality associated with the August 2003 heat wave raises fundamental questions about the concept of advance disaster planning and about the need to establish:

- alert procedures that are able to provide real-time information when calls to emergency departments or mortality reports increase to abnormal levels,
- an alert procedure based on meteorologic forecasts that makes it possible to anticipate by several days a risk of excess mortality associated with a heat wave and therefore provide additional time to plan effective prevention measures.
- a system to identify and describe the health and safety hazards (type, current or predicted, probability, scale of possible harmful effects).

Implementation of an effective combination of these three planning scales is a major public health objective. All institutions with relevant aims and skills must be recruited to this project, be strongly supported by public authorities, and demonstrate the reality and efficacy of their collaboration.

## Acknowledgments

We thank the four institutions that participated in this work: INSERM, INSEE, InVS and Météo-France. We also thank sincerely all those with whom we had direct contact within these institutions and who have efficiently and rigorously helped to provide the information on which this work is based: within INSERM 170-IFR69:J. Clavel, S. Bellec, C. Guihenneuc-Jouyaux and V. Lasserre – within INSERM-CépiDc-IFR69:F. Laurent, G. Pavillon, C. Jacquart, H. Lefèvre, M. Bovet, F. Péquignot, A. Le Toullec, M. Pauchard, as well all of the staff at CépiDc who helped prepare and code the data – within Inserm-DISC: N. Pinhas and D. Douguet – within INSEE:G. Desplanques, C. Beaume, F. Clanché, R. Merlen, D. Morineau, L. Doisneau – within InVS: G. Brucker, M. Ledrans, A. Le Tertre, M. Mettendorf,

S. Mediated – within Météo-France: P. Courtier, B. Rambaldelli, N. Bourdette, J. Manach. This work could not have been performed without the acceleration of death data by the mobilization of all of the district health departments and the vital statistics offices.

## References

Basu R, Samet JM (2002) Relation between elevated ambient temperature and mortality: a review of the epidemiologic evidence. Epidemiol Rev 24:190–202

Besancenot JP (2002) Vagues de chaleur et mortalité dans les grandes agglomérations urbaines. Environnement, Risques et Santé 4(1):229–240

Ellis FP, Nelson F, Pincus L (1975) Mortality during heat waves in New York City July, 1972 and August and September, 1973. Environ Res 10:1–13

Hemon D, Jougla E (2003) Surmortalité liée à la canicule d'août 2003 – rapport d'étape. Estimation de la surmortalité et principales caractéristiques épidémiologiques. Rapport remis au Ministre de la Santé et des Affaires Sociales et des PersonnesHandicapées le 25 septembre 2003: 59p.

InVS (20 août 2003) Impact sanitaire de la vague de chaleur en France survenue en août 2003. Rapport préliminaire. Département des Maladies Chroniques et Traumatismes – Département Santé Environnement.

Katsouyanni K, Trichopoulos D, Zavitsanos X, Touloumi G (1988) The 1987 Athens heat wave. Lancet 2:573

Météo-France (28 août 2003) Eléments climatologiques sur l'année 2003, conséquence du réchauffement global pour le climat de la France

MMWR (1994) Heat-related deaths – Philadelphia and United States, 1993–1994. MMWR Morb Mortal Wkly Rep 43:453–455

Oechsli FW, Buechley RW (1970) Excess mortality associated with three Los Angeles September hot spells. Environ Res 3:277–284

Rooney C, McMichael AJ, Kovats RS, Coleman MP (1998) Excess mortality in England and Wales, and in Greater London, during the 1995 heat wave. J Epidemiol Community Health 52:482–486

Sartor F, Snacken R, Demuth C, Walckiers D (1995) Temperature, ambient ozone levels, and mortality during summer 1994, in Belgium. Environ Res 70:105–113

Smoyer KE (1998) A comparative analysis of heat waves and associated mortality in St. Louis, Missouri –1980 and 1995. Int J Biometeorol 42:44–50

Whitman S, Good G, Donoghue ER, Benbow N, Shou W, Mou S (1997) Mortality in Chicago attributed to the July 1995 heat wave. Am J Publ Health 87:1515–1518.

# The Oldest-Old: Emergence of a New Population

*Jean-Marie Robine*[1]

## Summary

Although we know that the number of nonagenarians and centenarians is rapidly increasing in low mortality countries, monitoring this development with accuracy remains difficult. Basic information on the number of centenarians comes from censuses. They make it possible to adjust annual population counts and to provide annual estimates of the number of centenarians, from which we can estimate the Centenarian Doubling Time (CDT). The registration of deaths, year after year, provides a much more accurate indication of the increase in the number of centenarians than do series of censuses. We propose that the Centenarian Rate (CR), i.e., the ratio of the number of centenarians to the number of people belonging to the same cohort – aged 60 years 40 years before – per 10,000 persons, allows us to assess the importance of the number of centenarians in many countries today with simple empirical data.

## Introduction

Although, we know that the number of centenarians is increasing substantially in low mortality countries (Vaupel and Jeune 1995), we still have problems monitoring this phenomenon accurately. Japanese (Robine and Saito 2003; Robine et al. 2003) and French data suggest an acceleration in the rate of increase in centenarians, whereas data from some other countries suggest a rapid deceleration, even revealing a decrease in the number of male centenarians. For instance, in Denmark and the Netherlands, the number of centenarians decreased by 26 and 22%, respectively, for males and increased by only 53 and 55%, respectively, for females in the 10 years from 1990 to 2000.

In this paper, we study the emergence of centenarians in developed countries for which we have been able to gather long series of data (Robine et al., 2005). We use census data and annual population counts as well as mortality data. We introduce and compute the Centenarian Doubling Time (CDT) and various ratios such as the Centenarian Rate (CR). Eventually, we discuss the functional health status of this new segment of the population. The paper mainly deals with crude

[1] Inserm, Démographie et Santé, CRLC & Université de Montpellier 1, Centre de recherche de val d'Aurelle, 34298 Montpellier Cedex 05, France; e-mail: robine@valdorel.fnclcc.fr

Carey et al.
Longevity and Frailty

numbers. Its goal is to better describe the population of centenarians and this population's emergence in low mortality countries and to answer the following questions. Is the population of centenarians comparable from one country to another? Is the pattern of emergence unique to certain countries? What do we know about the heath status of the oldest-old populations?

## Census, annual population counts and death records

The basic information about the number of centenarians in a country is derived from censuses. Although the National Institutes of Statistics (NIS) and Census Bureaus are now attentive to the oldest-old, difficulties remain in properly enumerating them and official figures are still subject to debate in many countries. In France, for instance, the 1999 March census officially enumerated 11,593 centenarians: 1,476 males and 10,177 female; however, the population counts for January 1, 1999, after adjustment of the 1999 census, found only 885 males and 6,369 females, still a large number in comparison with the 1990 figures.[1] Indeed, the 1990 census had also enumerated too many centenarians: 5,081 persons; after adjustment of the 1990 census, the population counts for January 1, 1990, found only 3,760 centenarians – 470 males and 3,760 females. However, all the existing time series show a huge increase in centenarians enumerated from 1970 onwards. They also show a clear decreasing trend in the last decades of the 19th century and/or in the first decades of the 20th century and fluctuations in the 1950s or 1960s due to the combination of small numbers and difficulties in enumeration. These phenomena have been well illustrated by Bernard Jeune and his colleagues for Denmark, one of the European Nordic countries (Jeune 1995; Skytthe and Jeune 1995).

Censuses make it possible to adjust annual population counts and to provide an estimate of the number of centenarians each year. Generally, figures are given for persons aged 100 years and over. Thus, we have been able to gather long annual series for most Nordic and Western European countries, as well as for Japan. The number of recorded deaths of centenarians, on the other hand, only provides an indirect measure of the number of centenarians, since their death rate can change over time. Even with this limit, however, the registration of deaths, year after year, provides a much more accurate indication of the increase in the number of centenarians than does a series of censuses.

Figure 1 shows the fluctuations in the number of enumerated centenarians in Denmark from 1800 to 1930. The decrease in the number of centenarians from 1840 to 1900 probably can be explained by an improvement in the quality of statistics during the 19th century (Jeune 1995). Changes in borders during the 19th century and at the beginning of the 20th century can also explain part of the observed fluctuations in Denmark and other European countries. Figure 2 shows census data for the period 1860–1980 in four countries: Italy, Japan, Sweden and

[1] It seems that the figures given by the 1999 census for the population aged 100 years and over also comprised people in their 100th year, i.e., persons aged 99 years.

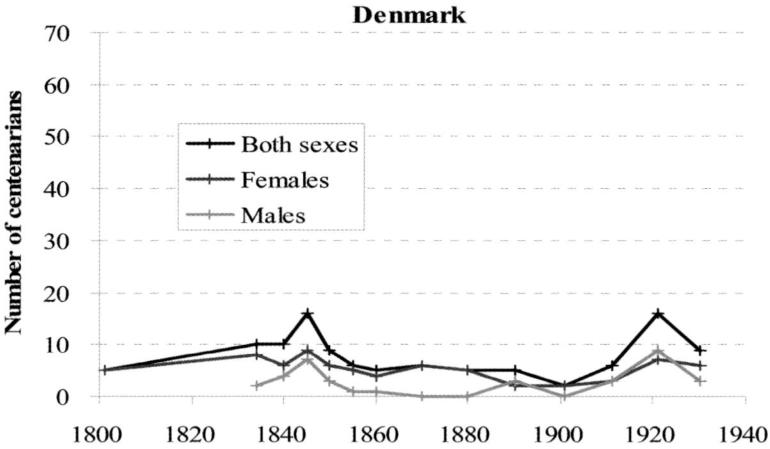


**Fig. 1.** Persons aged 100 years and over according to various censuses during the 19th and early 20th centuries in Denmark. Source: Data provided by Kirill F Andreev (2002). Source: ISTAT for Italy, Ministry of Health and Welfare for Japan, Statistics Sweden for Sweden and Office fédéral de la statistique for Switzerland. *From 1968 onwards, information is based on a register for Sweden

Switzerland. In Italy, the number of enumerated centenarians clearly decreased until 1931. In Japan, the first censuses showed fluctuations in the number of centenarians. In Switzerland, the number of enumerated centenarians remained extremely low during the first decades of the 20th century and fluctuated somewhat during the period 1930–1950. Looking at the four countries together, the increase appears exponential since at least the 1970s. However, in Sweden, the number of centenarians seems to increase sooner than in other countries, as early as the 1950s. The census series do not comprise enough points to allow a refined analysis of time trends; therefore, we move to annual estimations.

Figure 3 displays four of the longest annual series of population counts. Beyond a general increasing pattern, the increase in the number of persons aged 100 years and over seems to be stronger in Japan. The increase appears somewhat weaker in Sweden and England and Wales and much weaker in the Netherlands. In the last 10 years, there are striking differences in the increase in male centenarians between Japan, France and Switzerland on the one hand and Denmark and the Netherlands on the other. Denmark and the Netherlands appear to have experienced stagnation in the number of male centenarians compared to Japan, France and Switzerland, where there has been an acceleration of the increase. In between, Sweden, England and Wales display a more regular increase. Behind fluctuations due to small numbers, Norway resembles Sweden, England and Wales during the last 10 years.

In all countries, the number of deaths recorded each year has increased regularly since the 1950s (see Fig. 4) without significant fluctuations, contrary to population data provided by the censuses in the 1950s and 1960s. Interestingly, Figure 4 shows a decrease in the number of deaths of centenarians in the first

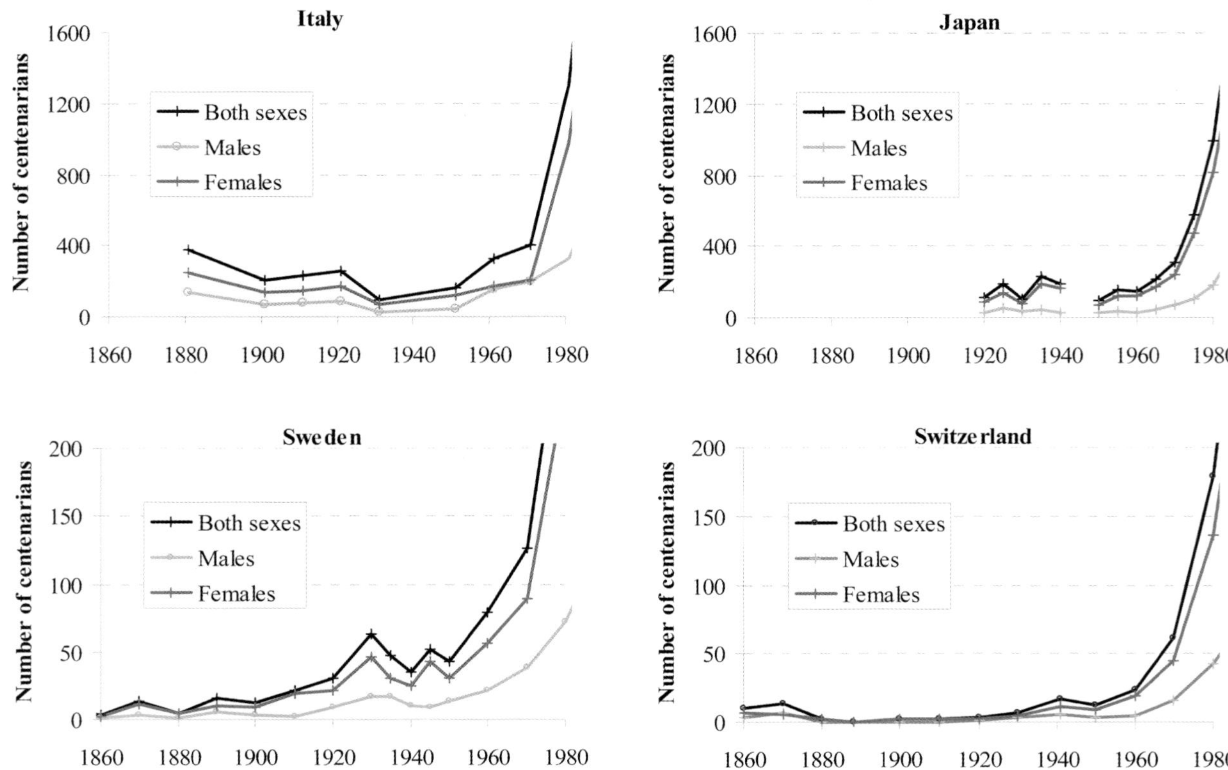


**Fig. 2.** Persons aged 100 years and over according to various censuses for the period 1860–1980 in four countries: Italy, Japan, Sweden* and Switzerland. Source: ISTAT for Italy, Ministry of Health and Welfare for Japan, Statistics Sweden for Sweden and Office fédéral de la statistique for Switzerland. *From 1968 onwards, information is based on a register for Sweden.

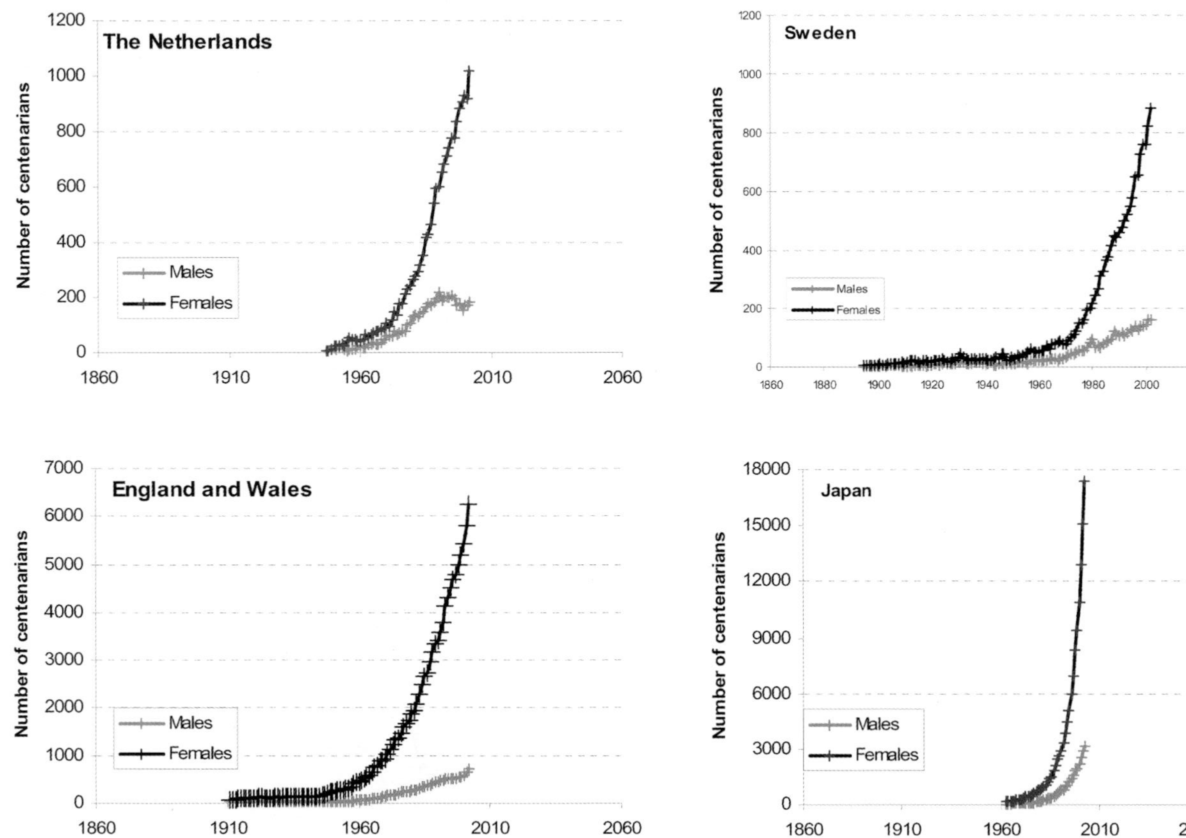


**Fig. 3.** Persons aged 100 years and over, by sex, according to annual population counts for the period 1860–2003 in four countries: the Netherlands (1947–2002), Sweden (1895–2002), England and Wales (1911–2002) and Japan (1963–2003).

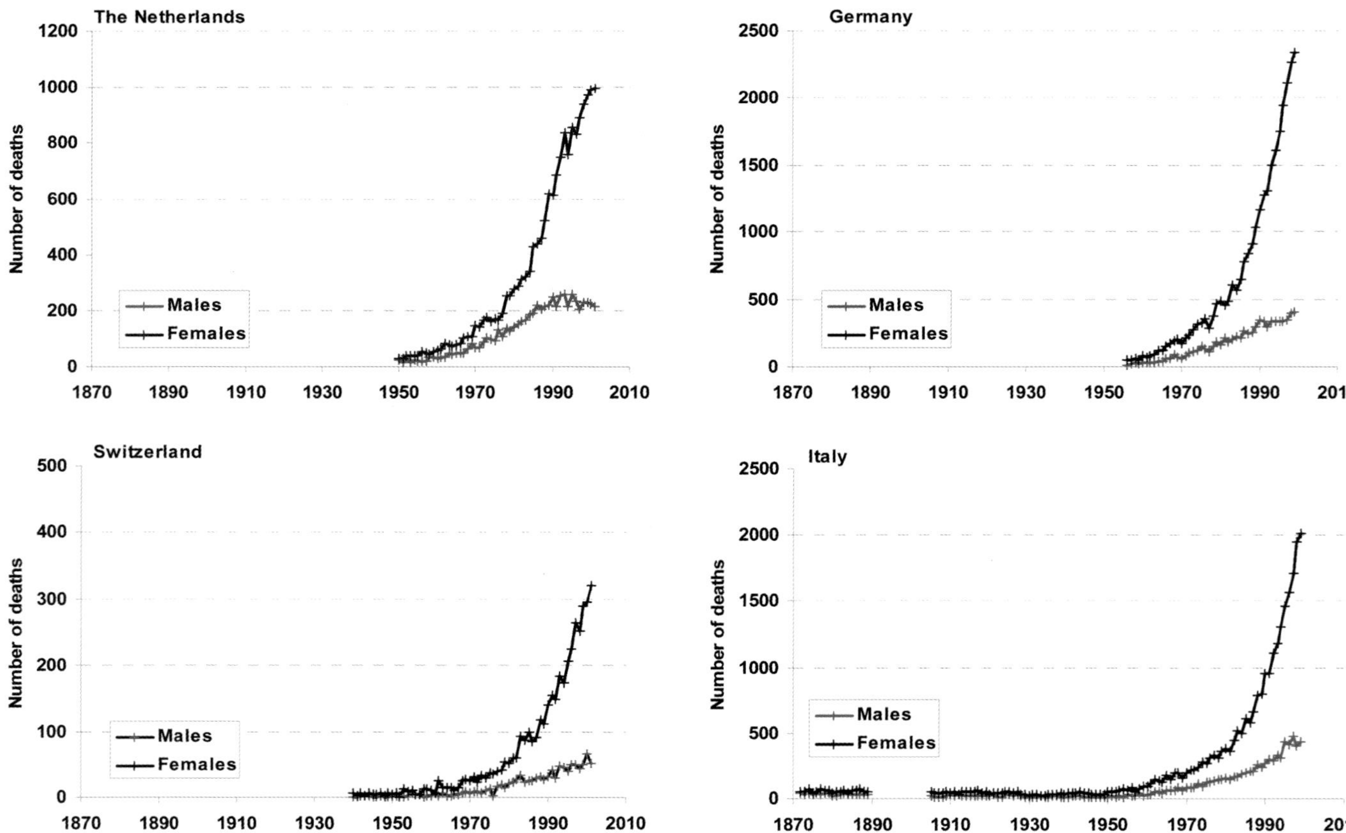


**Fig. 4.** Number of deaths of persons aged 100 years and over, in four countries: the Netherlands (1950–2001), Germany (1956–1999), Switzerland (1940–2001) and Italy (1872–1999). For the Netherlands, data are for deaths of persons aged 99 years and over. Source: Centraal Bureau voor de Statistiek, CBS for the Netherlands, Human Mortality Database for Germany, Office fédéral de la statistique for Switzerland, Ministry of Health and Welfare for Japan, and ISTAT for Italy,

half of the 20th century in Italy. All together, the data suggest that the number of centenarians regularly increased in low mortality countries since the 1950s in a much smoother way than is suggested by the various censuses, except in Japan, for which the increase started 10 to 20 years later. In recent years, divergent trends have appeared between the countries, especially for males. The mortality data clearly confirm this divergence.

## The Centenarian Doubling Time and the Centenarian Rate

Using the population counts, we can estimate the Centenarian Doubling Time (CDT). Previous work has suggested that the number of centenarians has doubled every 10 years in low mortality countries since the 1960s (Vaupel and Jeune 1995). However, recent work has shown that, in fact, the Centenarian Doubling Time is shortening for females in Japan (Robine et al. 2003) and France, whereas there is no change in England and Wales (Robine and Jagger 2003). The CDT is built on the annual rate of increase in the number of centenarians. After computing the annual rates of increase, we modelled the observed rates with linear interpolation to eliminate annual fluctuations and retain only the time trends. Then, using the standard formula to compute the population doubling time according to an exponential model, we computed the CDT from the interpolated values. The annual rates and the linear interpolations for six countries are displayed in Figure 5 and the corresponding CDT is shown in Figure 6.

Even with large fluctuations in small countries such as Denmark, the Netherlands, Sweden and Switzerland compared with England and Wales, Figure 5 shows clear time trends in the annual rate of increase in the number of centenarians. Three patterns emerge: the long-term trend clearly increases in France and Switzerland. It varies little in England and Wales and Sweden and clearly decreases in Denmark and the Netherlands. Figure 5 also shows that annual fluctuations diminish through time, especially in the smallest countries. However, compared to others, France displays relatively large fluctuations in recent years.

The corresponding CDT (Fig. 6) is consequently decreasing in France and Switzerland, varying little in England and Wales and Sweden, and increasing in Denmark and the Netherlands.

For the most recent years (see Table 1), the CDT in France has fallen to 7.5 and 5.3 years for females and males, respectively, as part of a decreasing trend. In Switzerland, it has fallen to 6.6 and 7.7 years for females and males, respectively, and in Japan to under five years for females; in both countries this is part of a decreasing trend. However, in England and Wales, the trend appears to be increasing, reaching 14.9 for females and 17.5 years for males. In Japan, it is more than six years for males, with a slightly increasing trend also. For females, the CDT is more than 17 years in Denmark and the Netherlands and close to 30 years in Norway, with predominantly increasing trends. For males, the CDT is close to 60 years in Norway in the most recent year and is infinite in Denmark and the Netherlands.

Figure 7 compares, for females, the rate of increase in the number of deaths and in the number of persons aged 100 years and over, in two countries: Japan,

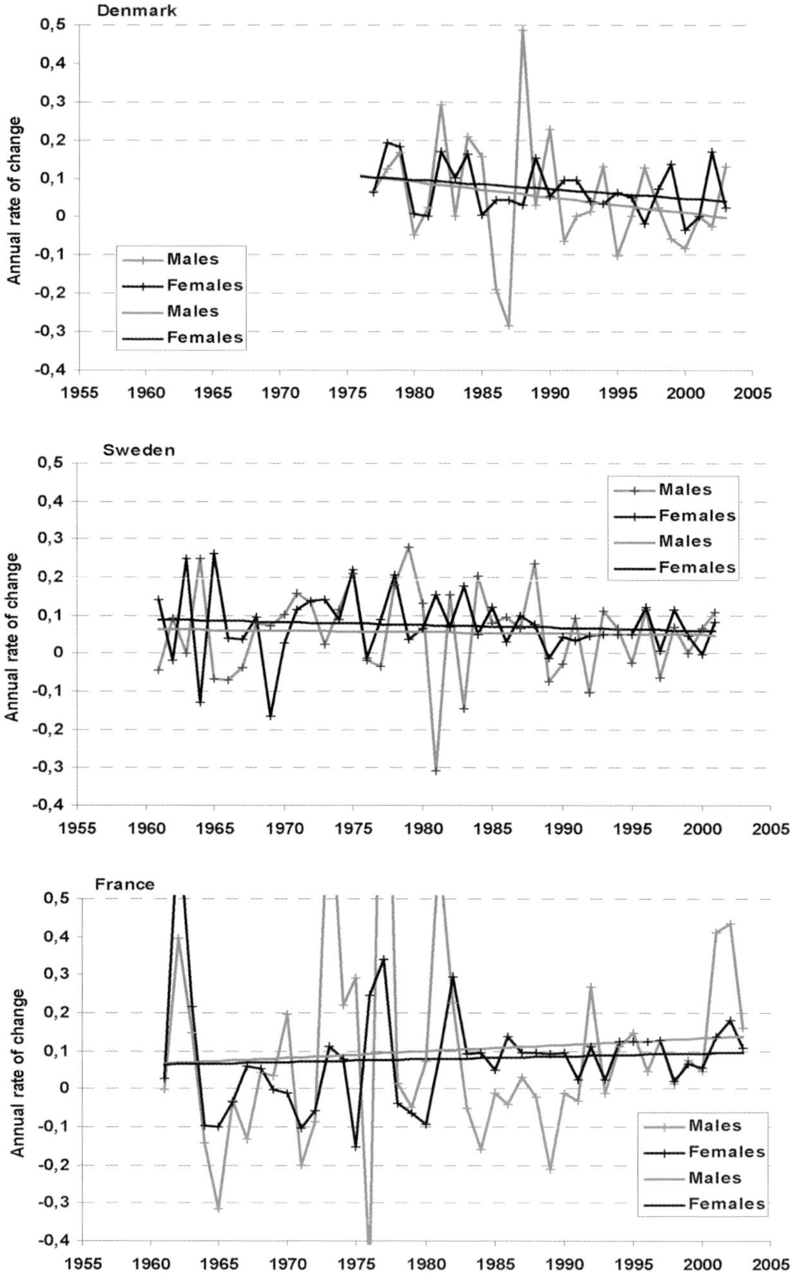


**Fig. 5.** Annual rate of change in the number of persons aged 100 years and over, by sex, according to the annual population counts – and linear interpolations – for the period 1960–2003 in six countries: Denmark (1976–2003), the Netherlands (1960–2002), Sweden (1960–2002), England and Wales (1960–2002), France (1960–2003) and Switzerland (1960–2001). For Switzerland, data are for persons aged 99 years and over.

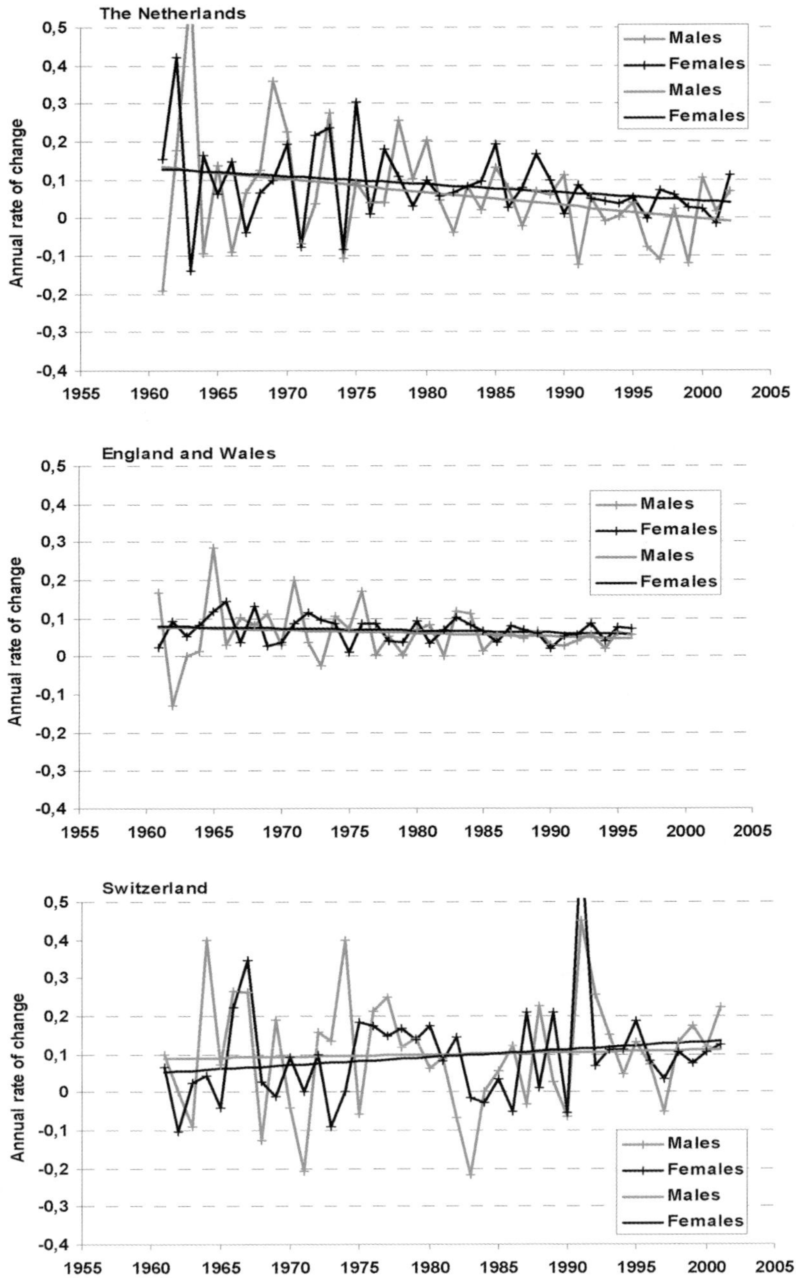


Fig. 5. *Continued*

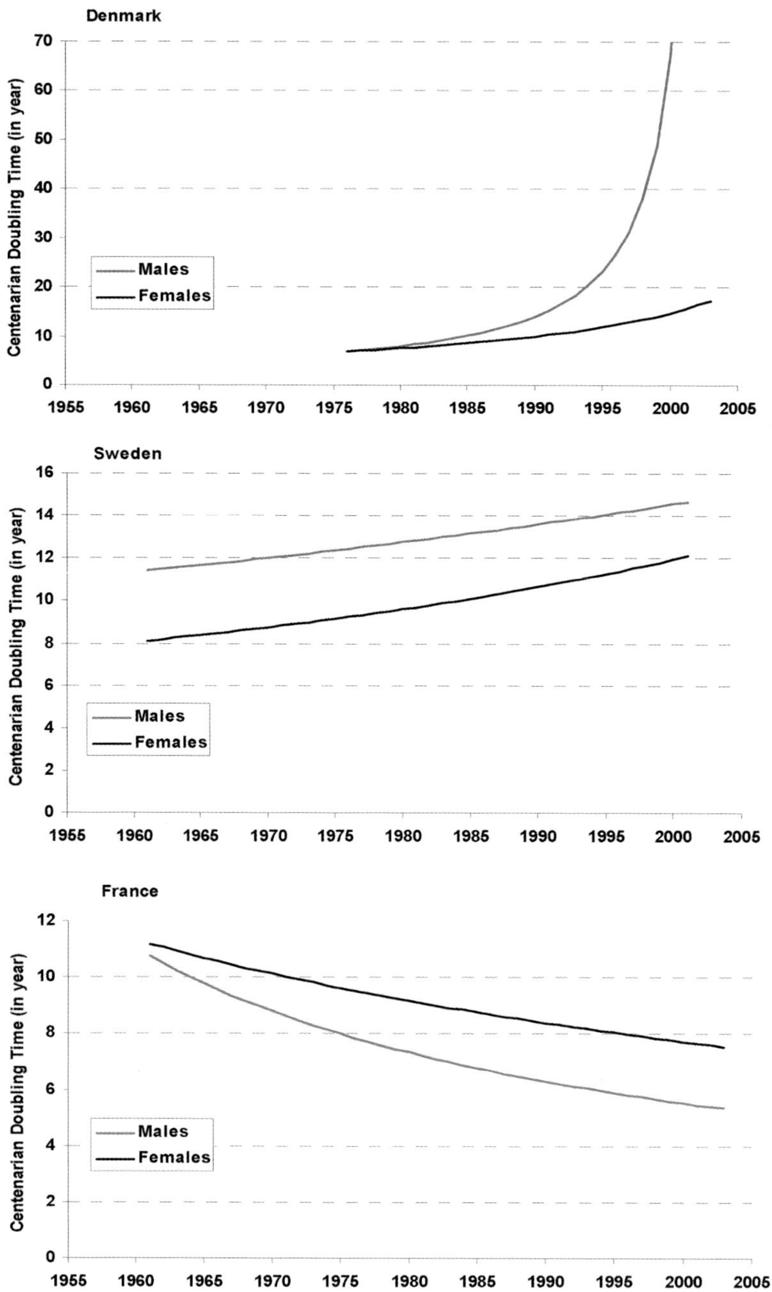


**Fig. 6.** Centenarian Doubling Time (CDT) by year for the period 1960–2003, by sex, in six countries: Denmark (1976–2003), the Netherlands (1960–2002), Sweden (1960–2002), England and Wales (1960–2002), France (1960–2003) and Switzerland (1960–2001). For Switzerland, data are for persons aged 99 years and over.

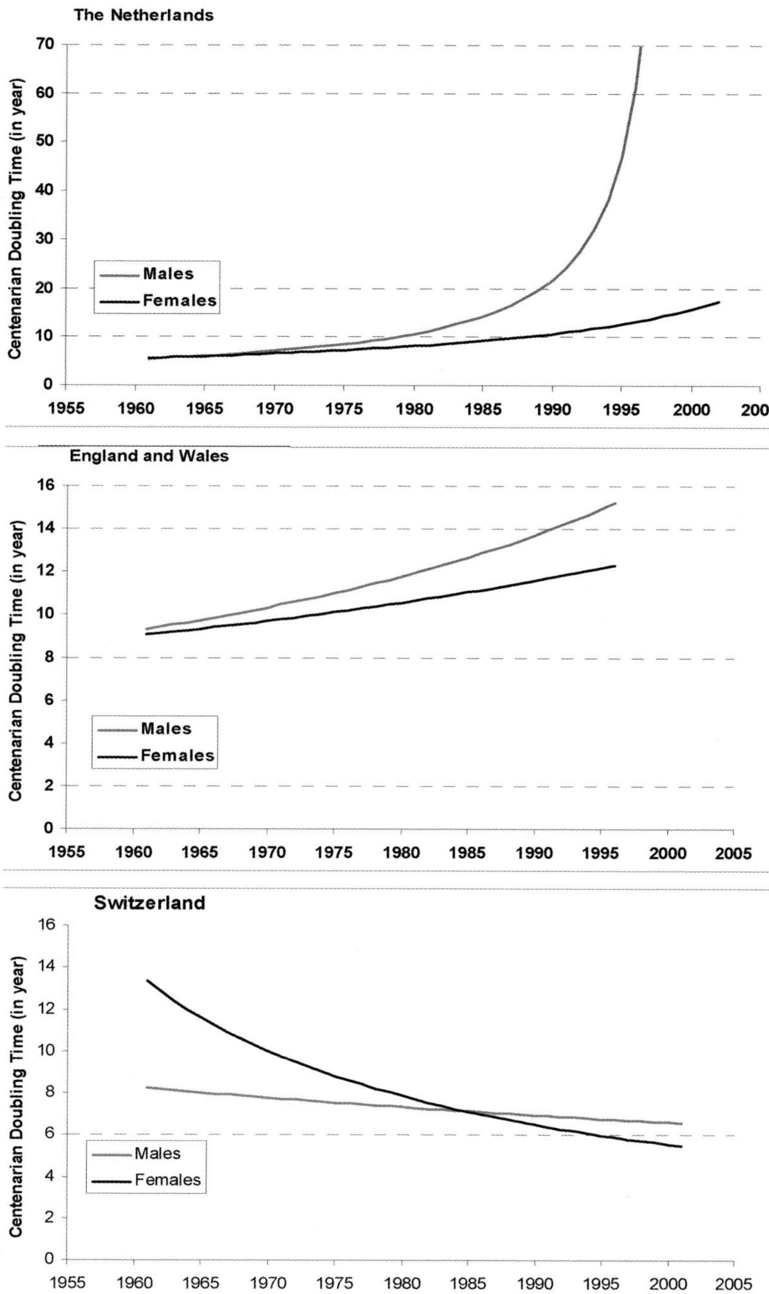


**Fig. 6.** *Continued*

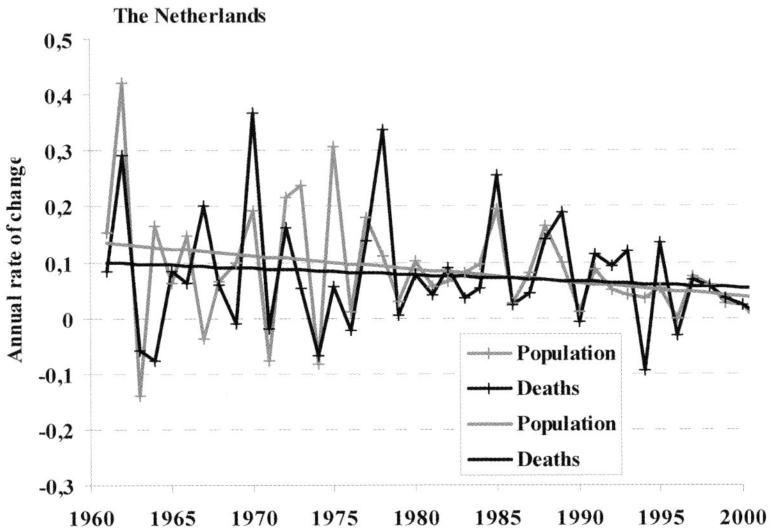


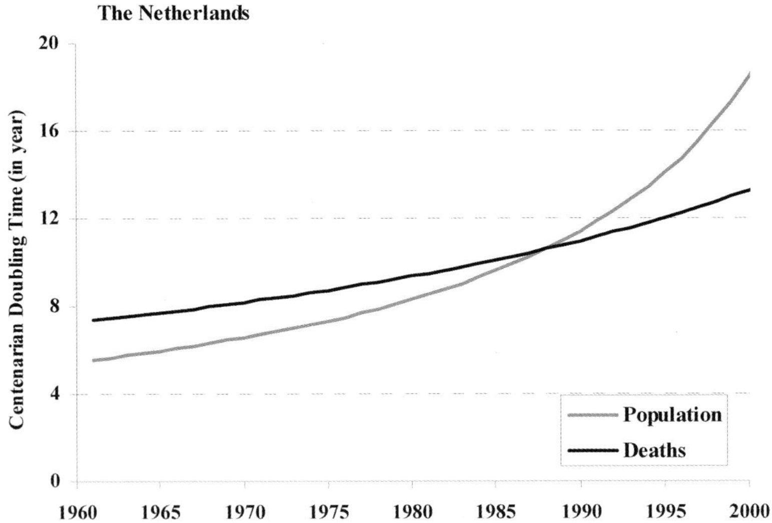


**Fig. 7.** Annual rate of increase in the number of deaths and in the number of persons aged 100 years and over – and linear interpolations (upper panel) – and Doubling Time (lower panel) for females in the Netherlands (1960–2001) and Japan (1963–2000). For the Netherlands, data are for deaths of persons aged 99 years and over.

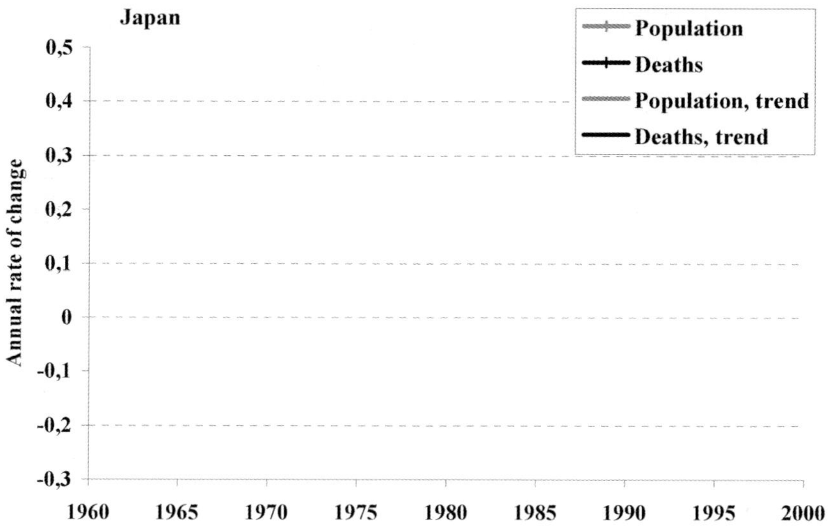


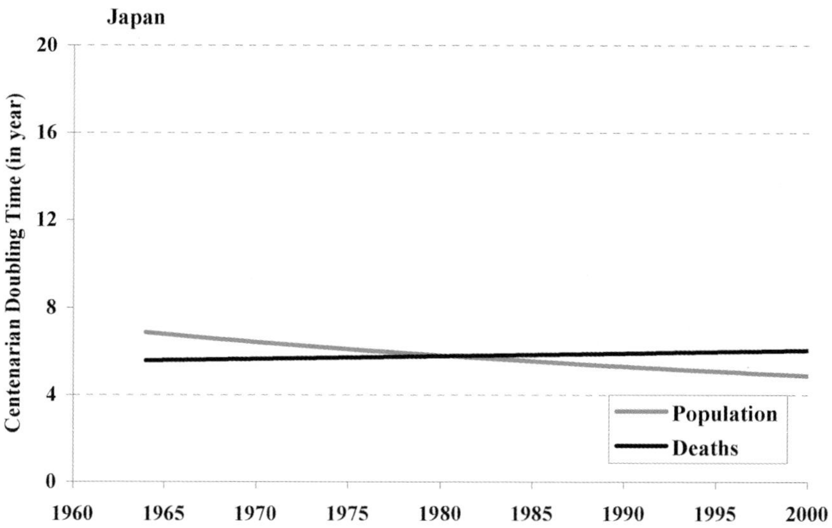


**Fig. 7.** *Continued*

**Table 1.** Centenarian Doubling Time (CDT) for the most recent years in eight countries

| Countries* | 2000 | 2001 | 2002 | 2003 |
|---|---|---|---|---|
| Male | | | | |
| France | 5.5 | 5.5 | 5.4 | 5.3 |
| Japan | 6.5 | 6.6 | 6.7 | 6.8 |
| Switzerland | 6.6 | 6.6 | – | – |
| Sweden | 14.6 | 14.7 | – | – |
| England and Wales | 16.8 | 17.1 | 17.5 | – |
| Norway | 40.5 | 45.8 | 52.5 | 61.7 |
| Denmark | 67.5 | 110.2 | 302.5 | infinite |
| Netherlands | infinite | infinite | infinite | – |
| Female | | | | |
| Japan | 4.8 | 4.7 | 4.7 | 4.7 |
| Switzerland | 5.5 | 5.5 | – | – |
| France | 7.7 | 7.7 | 7.6 | 7.5 |
| Sweden | 12.0 | 12.1 | – | – |
| England and Wales | 14.4 | 14.6 | 14.9 | – |
| Denmark | 14.8 | 15.5 | 16.4 | 17.3 |
| Netherlands | 15.7 | 16.5 | 17.4 | – |
| Norway | 22.6 | 24.6 | 27.0 | 29.9 |

*Countries are ranked according to their CDT in 2000 and 2001

which displays one of the strongest increases in the number of centenarians, and the Netherlands, which displays one of the weakest. As expected, the rate of increase in the number of persons aged 100 years and over increases in Japan, whereas the rate of increase in the number of deaths slightly decreases. Accordingly, the doubling time clearly declines for the number of female centenarians in Japan whereas the doubling time for the number of deaths slightly increases. These divergent trends are due to the fall of mortality among the Japanese centenarians (Robine et al. 2003). In contrast, in the Netherlands, the rates of increase in the number of centenarians and in the number of deaths decrease. As a result, the doubling time significantly increases and is faster for the number of centenarians than for the number of deaths. These trends are due to the increase in mortality among the Dutch oldest-old (Nusselder and Mackenbach 2000; Janssen et al. 2003). Consequently, for female centenarians, the number of people increases slower than the number of deaths.

How can we interpret all these figures and trends? How can we assess the importance of the number of centenarians observed in a country when the sizes of the countries studied are quite different? Do the observed figures differ from those expected? What should we use as the reference population, the current population or the one 100 years ago at the time of the centenarians' birth? Intuitively, the ratio of the number of current centenarians to the number of births occurring one century earlier can be affected by migration into and out of the country. Indeed, the 20th century witnessed much migration in most of the countries studied. The ratio of the number of centenarians to the current population is, however, no better, for in both cases it is impossible to control for the migrations that have impacted the population and its structure between the birth of centenarians and their hundredth birthday.

Graziella Caselli suggests that we use the Centenarian Rate (CR), defined as the ratio of the number of centenarians to the number of people who were aged 60 years 40 years before, expressed per 10,000. The objective is to get an indicator that is comparable in time and space, making it possible to study changes over time and to establish international comparisons. For Caselli, taking the survivors at age 60 years as a reference reduces the impact of most of the perturbations related to migration (Robine et al., submitted for publication). In addition, the Swiss data suggest that this approach would reduce the variability surrounding the acquisition of nationality (Robine and Paccaud, 2005). Indeed, taking the number of individuals at age 60 as the denominator of the ratios eliminates many unwanted effects, such as those related to infant mortality – which was still important one century ago and varied widely from one country to another – and those related to migration and naturalization. On the other hand such a denominator retains most of the adult mortality. The assumption is that the number of centenarians in any country depends primarily on the number of individuals aged 60 years 40 years earlier and of the trajectories of mortality after this age. It is on this principle that the CR is built. Such a ratio should make it possible to correctly compare the number of centenarians in various countries where infant mortality more than one century ago, past migratory models and policies of naturalization could be very different, as in France, Italy or Japan.

Figure 8 displays chronological series of the CR in five countries. It clearly shows a general pattern through the 20th century. The centenarian rate regularly increases from about one centenarian in 1900 for 10,000 persons aged 60 years 40 years before (in 1860), such as in Switzerland, to 40 centenarians for males and 160 centenarians for females, respectively, around the year 2000, for 10,000 persons aged 60 years 40 years before. For females, all together the centenarian rate reaches 20 in the 1970s, 60 around the year 1990 and 160 around the year 2000. Three countries (France, Japan and Switzerland) seem to follow this general pattern exactly, whereas Denmark and the Netherlands diverge from it in the 1990s and show stagnation, at least until the first years of the 21st century. For males, all together the centenarian rate increases much more slowly, reaching 20 in the 1980s and 40 around the year 2000. Two countries follow this general pattern, Japan and Switzerland, whereas Denmark and the Netherlands clearly diverge from

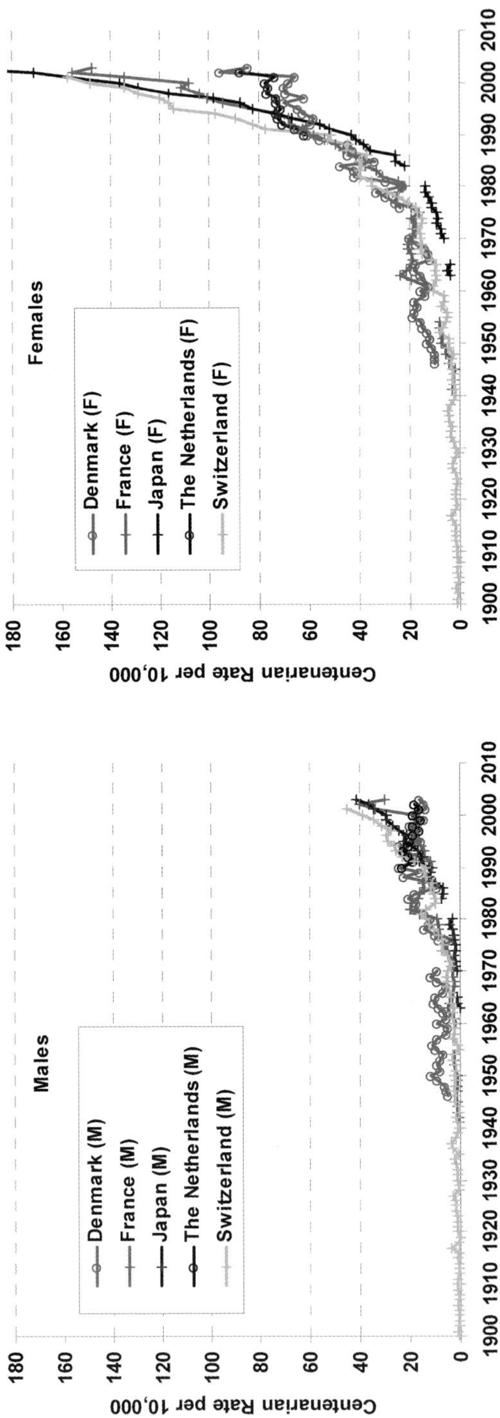


**Fig. 8.** Centenarian Rate in five countries: Denmark (1946–2003), France (1941–2003), Japan (1963–2003), the Netherlands (1990–2002) and Switzerland (1900–2001). M, males; F, females.

the pattern, first reaching a plateau in the 1980s (Denmark), and then decreasing in the 1990s. France appears in between: evolving like Denmark, reaching a plateau in the 1980s and in the beginning of the 1990s and then catching up with Japan and Switzerland around the year 2000. It is noteworthy that the increase in the CR starts later in Japan by comparison with the other countries, but Japan catches up with Switzerland in the late 1990s, at least for females.

## Discussion

What is the interest in studying the emergence of the population of centenarians, the crude figures and the pace of increase in low mortality countries? Why is the Centenarian Rate interesting? Why should we not be satisfied with death rates and the probabilities of surviving to age 100 from longitudinal life tables? Life tables are statistical models and are still difficult to complete for the oldest ages. On the other hand, crude figures on centenarians are now available in many countries, as are data on the population aged 60 years 40 years previously. The Centenarian Rate allows us to assess the importance of the number of centenarians in many countries today with simple empirical data, enabling a comparison of countries where the size of the birth cohorts, infant mortality, past migrations and policies of naturalization could vary widely.

When an accurate death rate at age 100 is available, it could, alongside infant mortality, allow us to monitor how a country protects its frailest citizens. In fact, mortality studies have shown that centenarians are extremely frail people, with a mortality almost doubling in winter by comparison with the summer months (Robine and Vaupel 2001; Robine and Saito 2003). The August 2003 heat wave in Europe demonstrated again this extreme vulnerability of the oldest-old to the climate. However, until we have such data, the CR provides the means to more accurately monitor trends in this new and frail segment of our population.

### What are the relationships between the CR and infant mortality?

One century ago, the infant mortality rate (IMR) was quite high and may have differently selected people surviving to age 60 in the 1960s, which in turn can explain the observed CR in 2001. Today, infant mortality is very low and varies little, but the IMR is still one of the most used indicators to assess the effectiveness and the equity of the health sector (Reidpath and Allotey 2003). Does the CR draw the same conclusion as the IMR on the effectiveness and the equity of the health sector to protect the most frail in the low mortality countries?

Table 2 shows the infant mortality rates, one century ago, in 1900 and 1901 and in 2000 for the 10 studied countries. The countries are ranked according to the IMR in 1900. This ranking significantly varies from the one we can get from CR. Infant mortality was clearly lower in Nordic countries one century ago and, obviously, the population aged 60 years in the 1960s was much less selected by infant mortality in Norway or in Sweden than in England, France or Germany. But there is no clear correlation between the IMR one century ago and the current CR

**Table 2.** Infant mortality per 1000, in 1900, 1901 and 2000, for 10 low mortality countries

| Countries[a] | 1900 | 1901 | 2000[b] |
|---|---|---|---|
| Norway | 86.3 | 87.5 | 3.8 |
| Sweden | 107.0 | 110.3 | 3.4 |
| Denmark | 128.9 | 134.3 | 5.3 |
| Japan | 155.0 | 149.9 | 3.9 |
| The Netherlands | 164.5 | 158.4 | 5.1 |
| Switzerland | 164.6 | 152.0 | 5.0 |
| England and Wales | 171.7 | 171.1 | 5.8 |
| Italy[c] | 174.1 | 166.3 | 4.6 |
| France | 185.2 | 167.0 | 4.4 |
| Germany | 229.0 | 207.0 | 4.4 |

[a] Countries are ranked according to the infant mortality rate in 1900, [b] Sources: INED, www.ined.fr, 2003, [c] ISTAT, 1975

(Spearman's coefficient of correlation = 0.43 between CR2001 and IMR1900 and 0.23 between CR2001 and IMR1901). In particular, Denmark and Japan, being ranked the lowest and highest, respectively, according to the CR in 2001, occupy an intermediate position for the IMR in 1900 and 1901.

In the same way, there is no clear correlation between the current IMR and the CR (Spearman's coefficient of correlation = –0.33 between CR2001 and IMR2000). In 2000, Sweden, Norway and Japan ranked among the best according to the IMR, with a rate lower than 4 per 1000, whereas Switzerland, the Netherlands, Denmark and England and Wales stood among the worst of this selection of low mortality countries, with a rate higher than 5 per 1000. It is clear that some countries with an enviable IMR, such as Norway or Sweden, have a quite low CR. On the other hand, some countries with a high CR, such as Switzerland, do not have such a good IMR. This absence of correlation between classic population health indicators, such as the IMR and the CR, should encourage use of the latter for assessing the equity of the health sector to the older population.

This study clearly showed that there was a general pattern of emergence of the oldest-old in the low mortality countries through the 20$^{th}$ century. The centenarian rate for 10,000 persons aged 60 years 40 years before increases from a value close to "no one" in 1900 to 40 for males and 160 for females around the year 2000. However, before the end of World War II, changes in CR are unnoticeable. A few countries, such as Japan or Switzerland, follow this general pattern of increase up to 2000, whereas some countries in northern Europe, such as Denmark and the Netherlands, clearly show stagnation in the 1980s and 1990s. Other European countries appear in between, such as England and Wales, Norway and Sweden.

France appears somewhat closer to Japan and Switzerland. What can explain these newly divergent trends among the low mortality countries at the turn of the 21$^{st}$ century? To go further, comparative studies of the mortality trajectories for the oldest-old are needed.

## Acknowledgment

This study was undertaken within the framework of the IUSSP Committee on Longevity and Health and involved many researchers who provided the data and participated in the analysis: Jean-Marie Robine (Health and Demography, University of Montpellier 1, France), Graziella Caselli (Department of Demography, University La Sapienza, Rome, Italy), Yasuhiko Saito (Nihon University, Tokyo, Japan), Carol Jagger (University of Leceister, England), Fred Paccaud (Institut Universitaire de Médecine Sociale et Préventive, Université de Lausanne, Switzerland), Frans van Poppel (Netherlands Interdisciplinary Demographic Institute NIDI, The Hague, Netherlands), Hans Lundström (Statistics Sweden, Stockholm, Sweden), Celvin NJ Ruisdael ( Stavanger, Norway) and James W Vaupel (Max Planck Institute, Rostock, Germany).

## References

Andrev KF (2002) Evolution of the Danish population from 1835 to 2000. Odense Monographs on Population Aging 9. Odense University Press.

Jansen F, Nusselder WJ, Looman CWN, Mackenbach JP, Kunst AE (2003) Stagnation in mortality decline among elders in the Netherlands. The Gerontologist 43(5):722–734.

Jeune B (1995) In search of the first centenarians. In: Jeune B, Vaupel JW (eds) Exceptional longevity: from prehistory to the present. Odense Monographs on Population Aging 2. Odense University Press.

Nusselder WJ, Mackenbach JP (2000) Lack of improvement of life expectancy at advanced ages in the Netherlands. Intl J Epidemiol 29:140–148.

Reidpath DD, Allotey P (2003) Infant mortality rate as indicator of population health. J Epidemiol Commun Health 57(5):344–346.

Robine JM, Vaupel J (2001) Supercentenarians, slower ageing individuals or senile elderly? Exp Gerontol 36:915–930.

Robine JM, Jagger C (2003) Acceleration of the rate of increase of centenarians: a comparison of England, France and Japan. PAA (au; please supply additional publication information paper presented at the annual meeting of the Population Association of America, 2003)

Robine JM, Saito Y (2003) Survival beyond age 100: The case of Japan. Pop Dev Rev 29(suppl):208–228.

Robine JM, Paccaud F (2005) Nonagerians and centernarians in Switzerland, 1860–2001: a demographic analysis. Epidemiol Community Health 59:31–37

Robine JM, Saito Y, Jagger C (2003) The emergence of extremely old people: the case of Japan. Exp Gerontol 38:735–739.

Robine JM, Caselli G (2005) Unprecedented increase in the number of centenarians. Genus, in press

Skytthe A, Jeune B (1995) Danish centenarians after 1800. In: Jeune B, Vaupel JW (eds) Exceptional longevity: from prehistory to the present. Odense Monographs on Population Aging 2. Odense University Press.

Vaupel JW, Jeune B (1995) The emergence and proliferation of centenarians. In: Jeune B, Vaupel JW (eds) Exceptional longevity: from prehistory to the present. Odense Monographs on Population Aging 2. Odense University Press.

# Subject Index